OSCEsmart

50 Medical Student OSCEs
in Psychiatry

Dr. Esha Abrol
Dr Michael Webb

Executive Consulting Editor:
Dr. Sam Thenabadu

Ordering Information: Quantity sales. Special discounts are available on quantity purchases by corporations, associations, and others. For details, contact the publisher at the address above.

Orders by UK trade bookstores and wholesalers please visit www.scowenpublishing.com

Although every effort has been made to check this text, it is possible that errors have been made, readers are urged to check with the most up to date guidelines and safety regulations.

The authors and the publishers do not accept responsibility or legal liability for any errors in the text, or for the misuse of the material in this book.

Publisher's Cataloging-in-Publication data : OSCEsmart 50 medical student OSCEs in Psychiatry.

Copyright © 2017 Simon Cowen Publishing

ISBN-10: 0-9985267-4-6
ISBN-13: 978-0-9985267-4-4

For our families...
The Amazing Abrol's and the Wonderful Webb's...
For which we owe absolutely everything.
Esha and Michael

'For Ammi, Molly, Reuben and Rafa - I.L.Y.T.T.M.'
Sam

CONTENTS

Message from the authors

Doctors of all seniorities can remember the stress of the OSCE but even more so the stress of trying to study and practice for the OSCEs. A multitude of generic undergraduate and postgraduate resources can be found on line but quality, quantity, and completeness of content can vary. The aim of the OSCESmart editorial team is to bring together specialty focused books that have identified 50 core stations encompassing the essential categories of history taking, examinations, emergency moulages, clinical skills and data interpretation with a strong theme of communications running through all the stations.

The combined experience of consultants, registrars and junior doctors to write, edit and quality check these stations, promises to deliver content that is appropriate to reach a standard we would expect of new junior doctors entering their foundation internship years and into core training. It is important to know that these stations are all newly written and based at the level of clinical competencies we would expect from these grades of doctors. Learning objectives exist for undergraduate curricula and for the foundation years, and the scenarios are based and written around these. What they are not, are scenarios that have been 'borrowed' from any medical school.

Preparation is the key to success in most things, but never more so than for the OSCEs and a candidate that hasn't practised will soon be found out. These books will allow you to practice relevant scenarios with verified checklists to learn both content and the generic approach. The format will allow you to practice in groups with one person being the candidate, one the actor and one the examiner. Each scenario finishes with three learning points. Picture these as are three core learning tips that we would want you to take away if you had only a couple of days left to the exam. These OSCE scenarios promise to be a robust revision aide for the student looking to recap and consolidate for their exams, but equally importantly prepare them for life in clinical practice.

I am immensely proud of this OSCESmart series. I have had the pleasure of working with some of the brightest and most dynamic young clinicians and educators I know, and I am sure you will find this series covering the essential clinical specialties a truly robust and invaluable companion in those stressful times of revision. I must take this opportunity to thank my colleagues for all their hard work but most of all to thank my wonderful wife Molly for her unerring love and support and my sons Reuben and Rafael for all the joy they bring me.

Despite the challenging times the health service finds itself in, being a doctor remains a huge privilege. We hope that this OSCESmart series goes some way to help you achieve the excellence you and your patients deserve.

Best of luck, Dr Sam Thenabadu

Introduction to OSCE Smart in Psychiatry

ED, General Practice, Surgery, Orthopaedics... There is not one setting in modern day medicine which is exempt from psychiatric presentations. Whether you are seeing an elderly patient who has stopped taking their medication since the death of their partner, or a young girl who has overdosed in the emergency department, psychiatry is everywhere. This purpose of this book is to provide medical students with a psychiatric toolkit that will not only be useful in exam preparation, but also as you begin your career as a foundation doctor.

Psychiatric patients can be agitated, aggressive, demanding, and difficult to deal with. They test not only your clinical acumen, but also challenge your communication, empathy, conflict resolution and risk assessment skills. These are vital parts of the 'hidden curriculum' at medical school, and are vital in the armoury of any foundation doctor.

This book has been designed for a group of three students practicing OSCES, who rotate the role of actor, examiner, and candidate. There is so much learning to be gained from playing each of these roles, whilst covering a breadth of psychiatric skills such as counselling, Mental State Examination's (MSE), SBAR handovers, history taking and DRABCDE assessments. We have included versatile and challenging cases that could be encountered anywhere and everywhere, such as performing a capacity assessment on a surgical ward, and assessing a victim of domestic violence.

We would like to extend a big thank you to each of co-authors (Priya, Sian, Mel, Matt N, Matt L, Juliet, Golnar, Shivanthi, Georgia and Chloe) for their hard work and dedication to this project, and for putting up with our pestering; draft, after draft, after draft! The combination of newly qualified foundation year doctors with core and higher psychiatric trainees, all with interests in medical education, allows this book to balance years of experience with an understanding of the current demands of medical school OSCEs.

Our final thanks go to our parents (Katharine, Nigel, Rummy and Vinay), who have always been there to celebrate our achievements and pick us up when we are down, and our supervisor and pal, Dr Sam Thenabadu, for his guidance, support and relentless positivity.

We hope that Esha's passion for mental health and wellbeing, and Mike's unwavering enthusiasm for teaching, have come across throughout this book.

We wish you the best of luck with your exams, training and future career.

Esha Abrol & Michael Webb

About the Authors

Dr Esha Abrol

MBBS BSc PgCert (Medical Education)

Esha graduated from UCL Medical School in 2014 with MBBS and a BSc in Neuroscience. She completed her foundation training in South Thames Foundation School (STFS) at Royal Surrey County Hospital and Princess Royal University Hospital, where she chaired the Junior Doctor Education Committee (JDEC) and received a certificate of merit for her contribution to teaching. She has taught on the Training to Teach (TtT) course, written SBAs for UCL Medical School, and been a virtual learning environment tutor for a group of Year 4 medical students. During her Foundation Year 2, she passed the Royal College of Physicians (RCP) & University College London (UCL) PgCert in Medical Education with Merit. She is currently an LAS Core Trainee in Psychiatry (CT1) working in Camden & Islington NHS Foundation Trust. She is extremely passionate about the mental health and wellbeing of her patients and is excited to pursue a career in this fascinating field.

Importantly, without the hard work, dedication, support and dependability, of her partner, Dr Michael Webb, this book would not have been possible. Together we make the perfect team.

Dr Michael Webb

MBBS BSc PgCert (MedEd)

Michael graduated with MBBS from UCL Medical School in 2014 with an intercalated BSc in Biochemistry and Medical Sciences. At UCL he established a keen interest in medical education working as a tutor in a variety of educational groups including Sexpression, UCL Peer-Assisted Learning Scheme and engaging in extra-curricular projects including the UCLU Medical society, and the 'Case of the Month' online tutoring team. He has since completed the foundation programme in South Thames Foundation school working in William Harvey Hospital, Ashford for his first year, and The Princess Royal University Hospital, Orpington for his second foundation year where he received a certificate of merit for his contributions to Undergraduate teaching program. In 2015 he attained a Post Graduate Certificate in Medical Education with Merit at the Royal College of Physicians and University College London. He presently works at the Royal Surrey County Hospital in Guildford as a Junior Clinical Fellow in Intensive Care which he hopes will provide a springboard to ACCS and establishing a Career in Anaesthetics and Intensive Care. He also has aspirations of continuing his passion in medical education through the diploma and Master's programmes in medical education.

He would personally like to thank his partner Dr Esha Abrol for her irreplaceable support and ambition throughout the production of this book, and beyond. This book serves as a testament that her talent and capabilities have no limits.

Dr Sam Thenabadu

MBBS MRCP DRCOG DCH MA Clin Ed FRCEM MSc (Paed) FHEA

Consultant Adult & Paediatric Emergency Medicine
Honorary Senior Lecturer & Associate Director of Medical Education

Sam Thenabadu graduated from King's College Medical School in 2001 and dual trained in Adult and Paediatric Emergency Medicine in London before being appointed a consultant in 2011 at the Princess Royal University Hospital. He has Masters degrees in Clinical Medical Education and Advanced Paediatrics.

He is undergraduate director of medical education at the King's College NHS Trust and the academic block lead for Emergency Medicine and Critical Care at King's College School of Medicine. At postgraduate level he has been the Pan London Health Education England lead for CT3 paediatric emergency medicine trainees since 2011. Academically he has previously written two textbooks and has published in peer review journals and given numerous oral and poster presentations at national conferences in emergency medicine, paediatrics, medical education and patient quality and safety.

He has an unashamed passion for medical education and strives to achieve excellence for himself, his colleagues and his patients, hoping to always deliver this through an enjoyable learning environment. Service delivery and educational need not be two separate entities, and he hopes that those who have had great teachers will take it upon themselves to do the same for others in the future.

Co-authors

Dr Priya Abrol MBBS BSc
Foundation Year 1 Doctor (FY1) - St Peter's Hospital, London

Dr Golnar Aref-Adib MBBS BMedSci PGDipCAT MRCPsych
Specialist Trainee (ST4) General Adult Psychiatry & NIHR Academic Clinical Fellow - UCL Division of Psychiatry, London and Camden & Islington NHS Foundation Trust, London

Dr Juliet Davidson MBBS BSc
Foundation Year 2 Doctor (FY2) - Brighton

Dr Sian L Holdridge MBBS BSc
Core Psychiatry Trainee (CT1) - London

Dr Melanie Knowles MBBS BSc
Core Psychiatry Trainee (CT2) - Barnet, Enfield and Haringey Mental Health Trust, London

Dr Matthew Loughran MBChB BSc (Hons)
Core Psychiatry Trainee (CT2) - Royal Free London NHS Foundation Trust, London

Dr Matthew L Naylor MBBS BSc
Foundation Year 2 Doctor (FY2) - Tunbridge Wells Hospital, Royal Tunbridge Wells

Dr Shivanthi Sathanandan MBBS BSc MRCPsych
Specialist Trainee (ST6) General Adult Psychiatry and Fellow at Practitioners' Health Programme - UCL Partners, London

Dr Elizabeth Templeton MBCHB (Hons)
Core Psychiatry Trainee (CT3) - Camden & Islington NHS Foundation Trust, London

Dr Chloe Wilkes BMBS BMedSci
Foundation Year 2 Doctor (FY2) - East Sussex

Abbreviations

AMHP: Approved Mental Health Professional
CMHT: Community Mental Health Team
ED: Emergency Department
LD: Learning disability
MHA: Mental Health Act
DSH: Deliberate Self-Harm
BPAD: Bipolar Affective Disorder (BPAD)
EUPD: Emotionally Unstable Personality Disorder (EUPD)
CBT: Cognitive Behavioural Therapy
FBC: Full Blood Count
U&Es: Urea & Electrolytes
LFTs: Liver Function Tests
AMU: Acute Medical Unit
MSE: Mental State Examination
BP: Blood Pressure
ECG: Electrocardiogram
GP: General Practice
A&E: Accident and Emergency
PALs: Patient Advice and Liaison service
DV: Domestic violence
SBAR: Situation, Background, Assessment, Recommendations

General Adult Psychiatry

1.1 "Bleeding gums"

Candidate's Instructions:

You are a foundation year doctor in a GP practice. A 45-year-old supermarket cashier called Annabel attends with bleeding gums from excessive tooth brushing. She is not previously known to the practice.

Please take a history from this patient. You have 7 minutes, after which you will be asked to summarise and provide a management plan.

Examiner's Instructions:

A 45-year-old supermarket cashier called Annabel has attended their GP surgery with bleeding gums from excessive tooth brushing. She is not previously known to the practice.

The foundation year doctor based at the practice has been asked to take a history from this patient, with a view to summarise the findings.

At 7 minutes, ask the candidate for a summary and ask the following questions:

- What do you think the most likely diagnosis is for this patient? (Obsessive Compulsive Disorder)

- What differential diagnosis would you consider?

- What would you like to include in your initial management plan?

Actor's Instructions:

Background
You are a 45-year-old supermarket cashier called Annabel. You have been forced to come to see your GP by your sister who is concerned about excessive tooth brushing. You brush your teeth approximately 20 times per day, and have been doing so increasingly for the past 6 months, but more so in the past 2 weeks.

Your behaviour
You are anxious, rubbing your hands, embarrassed to be there. You are keen for reassurance. You are generally cooperative, but you do not feel you need to seek any help yourself, and are looking at the door as you are eager to leave the consultation.

Your history of symptoms
You admit this is bizarre behaviour, but cannot help worrying. You have tried to take your mind off brushing your teeth, but nothing works. You feel the behaviour is justified by the "trillions of germs" in the environment that enter your body through your teeth. These are your own thoughts, and all started six months ago, when one of your friends fell ill after contracting a heart condition (infective endocarditis) secondary to a dental infection.

You have a ritual involving a specific order of turning the taps on, washing your toothbrush in a particular way 10 times, brushing your teeth for 5 minutes, followed by mouthwash. This ritual improves your anxiety levels momentarily. You try to resist repeating the rituals, but this is difficult.

On direct questioning about symptoms of anxiety, you acknowledge these symptoms in yourself. Much of this anxiety is centred around your job. Concerns have been raised by how long it takes you to check items customers have bought. You are worried you may lose your job, and feel guilty and hopeless. When it all becomes too much, you feel your heart racing, you feel clammy and get butterflies in your stomach.

You do not have any previous medical or psychiatric history. As a child, you wouldn't step on cracks or walk under ladders. You do not take any medication. When asked about allergies, you say you are allergic to the "pesky germs" in the environment. You live alone, but your sister lives nearby. There is no family history of mental illness. You do not drink alcohol or smoke, and have never taken illicit drugs.

Your mental state
Your symptoms "get you down" but you are not low all the time. You generally sleep OK" but often wake up with worry. Your appetite and energy levels are also "OK." Your ability to enjoy things is "normal."

Questions and actions
Throughout the consultation: Do you think something is wrong with me doctor?

Markscheme:

Task:	Achieved	Not Achieved
Introduces self and clarifies who they are speaking to		
Gains consent		
Establishes nature of obsessions (onset, thoughts, images, ruminations, doubts)		
Establishes nature of compulsions (counting, washing, checking, rituals)		
Asks about physical symptoms (palpitations, breathlessness, sweating, dizziness) and biological symptoms (sleep, appetite)	✓	
Elicits any triggers (friend who was in hospital)		
Asks about core depressive symptoms (low mood, anhedonia, fatigue)		
Asks about past psychiatric history		
Asks about past medical history		
Asks about social history (drug, alcohol, smoking, employment)		
Asks about personal history (childhood, relationships, school)		
Asks about family history, including specifically about mental health and suicide		
Asks about medication history including allergies		
Asks about forensic history		
Performs a risk assessment in a sensitive manner (self-harm and suicidal ideation)		
Reassures patient in non-judgmental way		
Summarises consultation concisely		
Provides suitable primary diagnosis and relevant differentials (e.g. OCD, adjustment disorder, panic disorder, obsessive personality disorder)		

Explains basic steps for management (reassurance, support, CBT, behaviour therapy, 'flooding technique,' SSRIs)		
Establishes rapport with patient		
Examiner's Global Mark	/5	
Actor / Helper's Global Mark	/5	
Total Station Mark	/30	

Learning points:

- Obsessions are one's own thoughts and can be repetitive, intrusive and unpleasant. Compulsions are used to neutralize or prevent obsessions.

- Depression is commonly seen alongside OCD and other anxiety disorders, it is important to ask screening questions about the three core symptoms of depression, including low mood, reduced energy and lack of interest, in every anxiety disorder.

- Demonstrating empathy and reassurance is key with an anxious patient. Offering to bring the patient back in a week's time, perhaps with their sibling or carer, will signify this.

1.2 "Don't make me go back"

Candidate's Instructions:

You are a foundation year doctor in a GP practice. A 30-year-old flower shop owner called Ashleigh has attended the GP surgery due to always feeling on edge.

Please take a history from this patient. At 7 minutes you will be stopped to summarise your findings, investigation and management plan.

Examiner's Instructions:

A 30-year-old flower shop owner called Ashleigh has attended the GP surgery due to flashbacks, nightmares and feeling always on edge.

The foundation year doctor based at the practice has been asked to take a history from this patient, with a view to summarise the findings coherently.

Pay particular attention to the candidate's interaction with the timid, anxious patient.

At 7 minutes, ask the candidate to summarise the case, and ask the following questions:

- What do you think the most likely diagnosis is for this patient? (Post Traumatic Stress Disorder)

- What differential diagnosis would you consider?

- What would you like to include in your initial management plan?

Actor's Instructions:

Background
You are a 30-year-old flower shop owner called Ashleigh who was a victim of an attack 6 months ago.

Your behaviour
You are anxious, tearful, tremulous and restless. You are quiet, and do not volunteer any information unless specifically asked. When talking about the incident, you become very upset and angry.

Your history of symptoms
6 months ago, you were getting ready to close your flower shop with a co-worker at approximately 2330. Suddenly, a gang of three men in Halloween-style masks came into the store armed with knives. They grabbed you and your co-worker from behind, and demanded you to empty the till. Your co-worker shouted for help, and was subsequently beaten to the ground until they lost consciousness. You thought you were going to die. The men then emptied the till and then left abruptly as police sirens became audible in the distance, while you lay on the floor petrified.

Your co-worker made a good recovery, but after about one month, you became increasingly irritable, low in mood and anxious. You have lost your appetite, and 1 stone in weight over last 2 months. You are reluctant to see friends or go to social events. You cannot concentrate. This has been worsening of late, and you cannot sleep due to vivid nightmares of the event. You wake up sweating, shouting, and cannot get back to sleep. When you think about the events of that night, you feel as if you were there, with the same fear and horror. You feel panicked if doors slam unexpectedly. You look over your shoulder constantly, especially in busy, crowded places. You have not been back at work since the event, and avoid the whole area. Your passion for your flower business has completely diminished. You feel guilty that your co-worker was more badly injured than yourself.

You do not have any past medical history. You took a paracetamol overdose when you were 25 when your boyfriend split up with you, but have been since "signed off" by the mental health services. You do not take any medication but you are allergic to Trimethoprim. You live with your husband, who works away a lot. You find it difficult to share your feelings with your husband. There is no family history of mental illness. You have two younger brothers who both have young families. You were never the brightest student, and left school at 16 to start your own business. You were verbally bullied when you started secondary school for being the tallest girl in your class.

You do not smoke, and have never tried drugs. You normally drink socially but have started drinking daily for the past month; up to one bottle of wine per day to "help numb my feelings."

PTSD STATION OSCE – "Don't make me go back"

Task:	Achieved	Not Achieved
Introduces self		
Clarifies who they are speaking to and gains consent		
Elicits history of the traumatic event in a concise manner (nature, onset, triggers, timing, exacerbating factors)		
Establishes timing of symptoms (within 6m and present for more than 1m)		
Elicits re-experiencing, avoidance behaviour		
Asks about arousal and anxiety symptoms		
Asks about physical symptoms (palpitations, breathlessness, sweating, dizziness) and biological symptoms (sleep, appetite)		
Asks about past psychiatric history		
Asks about past medical history		
Asks about social history (drug, alcohol, smoking and employment)		
Asks about personal history (childhood, school, relationships)		
Asks about family history, including specifically about mental health and suicide		
Asks about medication history including allergies		
Performs a risk assessment in a sensitive manner		
Summarises consultation concisely		
Provides appropriate primary and differential diagnoses (PTSD, panic disorder, acute stress reaction, adjustment disorder, substance misuse)		
Explains basic steps for investigation (rule out organic causes, bloods e.g. TFTs, urine drug screen)		
Explains basic steps for management supportive management, coping strategies, CPN referral, CBT, eye movement desensitization reprocessing (EMDR), second-line medications such as paroxetine or mirtazapine)		

Establishes rapport		
Non judgmental approach		
Examiner's Global Mark	/5	
Actor / Helper's Global Mark	/5	
Total Station Mark	/30	

Learning Points

- A useful mnemonic to keep in mind when taking a PTSD history is 'TRAUMA':
    - **T**raumatic event
    - **R**e-experiencing (nightmares, flashbacks, memories, images),
    - **A**voidance and emotional numbing
    - **U**nable to function in social, occupational and interpersonal domains
    - **M**onth or more of symptoms
    - **A**rousal symptoms such as startle, irritability and hypervigilance.
- Think broadly about this patient, although PTSD is the most likely diagnosis, think about why this is not an acute stress reaction, adjustment disorder, substance misuse, or organic such as head injury.

- Patients with PTSD are extremely vulnerable. After establishing the history, always think about co-morbid depression, drug-alcohol abuse, and suicidality.

1.3 "I don't know, I'm not a doctor"

Candidate's Instructions:

You are a foundation year doctor based in the psychiatric outreach assessment clinic. Winnie, a 55-year-old-female, has been referred by her GP as she is extremely troubled by a multitude of different symptoms, despite normal test results and discharge from several specialist doctors.

Please take a history from this patient. You will be stopped after 7 minutes to provide a differential diagnosis and initial management plan.

Examiner's Instructions:

A 55-year-old female, Winnie, has been referred by her GP for a psychiatric opinion. The GP is concerned about an underlying somatoform disorder. Winnie has had multiple investigations (CT, MRI, PET scan) but still attends her GP frequently with different signs and symptoms that do not fit any recognisable diagnosis.

The foundation year doctor based in the psychiatric outreach assessment clinic has been asked to take a history from this patient. Please stop the candidate at 7 minutes and ask them to summarise the findings to the consultant psychiatrist and provide an initial management plan.

Actor's Instructions:

Background:
You are a 55-year-old single female called Winnie. You report a number of different symptoms such as abdominal pain, headaches, lethargy, dizziness and flushing, which have been changing and evolving over time. You are worried about a serious underlying condition.

Your behaviour:
You are anxious, fidgety and concerned about your symptoms. You don't understand why you have been sent to a psychiatrist but you are happy to discuss your symptoms.

Your history of symptoms:
You have been visiting the GP at least once per week per the past 2 years. You have had multiple investigations, including head and body imaging (CT, MRI, PET scan). You have been seen by lots of different specialists (rheumatologist, neurologist, endocrinologist, gynaecologist, gastroenterologist, ear nose and throat specialist), both on the NHS and privately.

You are not reassured by the negative results and think that doctors are missing something. You don't know exactly what could be wrong because: "I don't know I'm not a doctor!" You keep a notebook with you at all times detailing your blood pressure and heart rate fluctuations at different times of the day and other symptoms you might be experiencing. You record this using your personal blood pressure measuring device which you bought on the internet.

You have no known physical health problems, and have never had contact with psychiatric services previously. You do not take any regular medications, but you do take some herbal multivitamins from the internet. You do not have any siblings. Growing up, your mother was frequently in and out of hospital and had number of physical illnesses, including diabetes and multiple sclerosis. As a result, you often had to miss social activities to help your mum attend appointments or to do the housework.

You are currently working as a call centre advisor, but feel that your boss is not being supportive as she has spoken to you sternly about the number of sick days you have taken over the past year (at least 5 per month). You worry you might be fired.

You admit to feeling anxious and depressed over the last 6 months and have been drinking 3 large glasses of wine per night. You have never used illicit drugs or smoked.

Your mental state:
You sleep well and your appetite has not changed. You deny hallucinations or delusions. You have no self-harm or suicidal thoughts.

SOMATOFORM DISORDER STATION – "I don't know, I am not a doctor"

Task:	Achieved	Not Achieved
Introduces self		
Clarifies who they are speaking to and gains consent		
Explores nature, duration and frequency of multiple changing physical symptoms		
Asks about frequency of GP attendance and contact with specialist		
Asks whether the patient is concerned about a specific diagnosis		
Explores reaction to negative results, and lengths they are willing to go		
Explores any specific triggers, trauma or psychosocial stressors that could have triggered reassurance seeking behaviour e.g. pending court case or job loss that could be perpetuating behaviour		
Asks about functionality – do symptoms impact on work or social life		
Asks about mood symptoms (low mood, anhedonia, fatigue, concentration levels, sleep, appetite)		
Asks about anxiety symptoms (psychological and physical)		
Asks about past psychiatric history		
Asks about past medical history		
Elicits medication history and asks about allergies		
Asks about family history, including specifically about mental health and suicide, family or childhood illness		
Asks about social history (alcohol, smoking, drugs, employment)		
Performs a risk assessment in a sensitive manner including suicidal thoughts or self-harm		
Summarises consultation concisely		

Provides appropriate diagnosis (somatisation) and differentials (conversion disorder, panic attack, hypochondriasis)		
Explains basic steps for management (reassurance, support, CBT, behaviour therapy, advice to reduce drinking offer referral to alcohol service)		
Non judgmental approach		
Examiner's Global Mark	/5	
Actor / Helper's Global Mark	/5	
Total Station Mark	/30	

Learning Points

- A somatoform disorder diagnosis is made in the presence of a history of at least two years of multiple and variable physical symptoms that cannot be explained by any discernable physical disorders. Repeated consultations and sets of investigations with multiple primary care and specialist doctors is not uncommon.

- Patients are typically not reassured by negative results or only reassured for a short period of time.

- It is important to differentiate somatoform disorders from conversion disorders. In a conversion disorder, patients are fixated on one or two specific diagnosis or body parts.

1.4 "He loves me do"

Candidate's Instructions:

You are a foundation year doctor on your community psychiatry placement. Your next patient is a 45-year-old female, Sophia, who has referred by her GP who is concerned about her behaviour.

Please perform a full Mental State Examination (MSE). Please do not take a history. You have 5 minutes to do this, after which you will be asked to present the MSE including relevant negatives, summarise and answer some questions.

Examiner's Instructions:

A 45-year-old woman called Sophia has been referred to a community psychiatrist by her GP who is concerned. The foundation year doctor has been asked to complete a Mental State Examination (MSE).

At 5 minutes, please ask the candidate the following:

1. Please present the MSE...
2. Please explain your risk assessment...
3. What do you think is the most likely diagnosis? (Delusional disorder, erotomania (De Clerambault Syndrome))

Actor's Instructions:

Background:
You are a 45-year-old woman called Sophia. You work as a secretary. For the past four months you have realized that Prince William is secretly in love with you and wants to have a relationship with you.

This is a Mental State Examination (MSE) station, so the candidate should not take a history. If they ask, you have no past medical or psychiatric history.

Your mental state:

MSE component	Description
Appearance and Behaviour	You look well, appropriately-dressed and well-kempt. You have normal energy levels and are high functioning. You engage well in the conversation. You have good eye contact. Your behaviour alters through the consultation: when discussing Prince William being in love with you, you become embarrassed and gush with excitement. When the candidate challenges this, you quickly adopt an angry and accusatory manner.
Speech	Your speech is normal in rate, tone and volume. Your speech becomes loud and fast when the candidate challenges Prince William being in love with you.
Mood	You are "fine". You are sleeping well with no changes in your appetite or energy levels. You would rate your mood as 5/10.
Thought	Thought process – the answers you give are all relevant and appropriate. You don't veer off the topic, or give incomprehensible responses. No-one is interfering with your thoughts. Thought content – you believe that Prince William is secretly love with you. He wants to be with you but doesn't know how to tell his wife, Kate Middleton, and, more importantly, the Queen. You are "certain" that this is true and get angry if anyone tells you otherwise. You have evidence in the form of love letters, messages, videos and hundreds of witnesses. Those that don't believe you are "just jealous". When you

	see William on the TV or in the press it confirms how much he loves you. You are excited to finally meet Prince William when he comes to inaugurate the new local hospital next week so that you can make your relationship public.
	You do not believe you have any special powers or abilities. You deny any strong religious beliefs or convictions.
Perception	You are not experiencing any illusions and you are not hearing voices, or seeing anything or anyone that is not there (hallucinations). You do not responding to external stimuli during the consultation.
Cognition	You have not been confused or disorientated at any point. You know who you are, where you are, and what time it is.
Insight	If asked whether you think that your delusion may not be based in reality, become adamant that Prince William loves you. This makes you angry and accusative towards the candidate and proves that they, like your friends and family who challenge you, are all just jealous. You do not think you are unwell and do not feel you need psychiatric attention or medication.
Risk	You do not have any thoughts of hurting yourself or anyone else. You do not carry weapons and have not engaged in any attempts to meet Prince William yet, but are planning to attend the inauguration of the local hospital next week so that he can declare his love to you. You are not sure if you will be able to control your emotions if this does not go to plan.

DELUSIONAL DISORDER MSE - HE LOVES ME DO

Task:	Achieved	Not Achieved
Introduces self		
Clarifies who they are speaking to and gains consent from patient		
Establishes rapport		
Elicits history of delusions in a concise and fluent manner		
Comments on Appearance (height, overweight/underweight, clothing, kempt/unkempt).		
Comments on Behaviour (distraction, fidgety, suspicious)		
Comments on Speech (rate/volume/tone)		
Comments on Objective Mood (low/Euthymic/Elated)		
Comments on Affect (reactive/Flat/Blunted)		
Comments on Subjective Mood (Sad, Hopeless, Happy, Optimistic).		
Comments on Thought Form (No disorder of thought form)		
Comments on Thought Content (erotomanic delusions about Prince William, strength of delusions).		
Comments on Visual hallucinations		
Comments on Auditory hallucinations		
Comments on cognition (Includes whether patient is orientated in time, place, and person)		
Comments on level of insight "do you think you are unwell?" "Do you think you need medication?"		
Enquires specifically about suicidal thoughts and risk		
Presents MSE concisely and fluently		

Performs a detailed risk assessment (including self-harm, suicide, stalking, harassment, harming others)		
Provides diagnosis and suitable differential (Delusional disorder, erotomania (De Clerambault Syndrome))		
Examiner's Global Mark	/5	
Actor / Helper's Global Mark	/5	
Total Station Mark	/30	

Learning Points

- Delusional disorder is a relatively uncommon disorder where the only clinical characteristic is a set or a single delusion. The delusions must be present for at least three months. If symptoms have been present for greater than 6 months, the outcome is often worse. Patients affected tend to have non-bizarre delusions with well preserved personal and social skills. This condition typically responds to antipsychotic medication.

- The delusions are often elaborate and systematised. Cognition and memory are intact, DSM- classifies delusional disorder into subtypes including; erotomanic (De Clarembault Syndrome), grandiose, jealous (Othello Syndrome) and persecutory.

- Differential diagnoses are wide, and may include:
  Schizophrenia
  Mood disorders with delusions
  Body Dysmorphic Disorder
  Obsessive Compulsive disorder
  Hypochondriasis
  Paranoid personality disorder
  Organic disorder- head injury, CNS infection, epilepsy.

1.5 "Feeling blue"

Candidate's Instructions:

You are a foundation year doctor on your GP placement. You are seeing your own patients this morning. The first patient is 52-year-old Roya.

Please take a history. You will be stopped after 7 minutes to summarise, and provide a differential diagnosis.

Examiner's Instructions:

A 52-year-old woman, Roya, has come into her GP surgery to discuss her mood. The foundation year doctor has been asked to take a history from her, followed by a summary and differential diagnosis based on the symptoms described.

Please stop the candidate at 7 minutes and ask them to summarise and state the differential diagnoses. Please prompt the candidate to justify the severity of the diagnosis (mild, moderate or severe) if they do not do so, and to explain why.

Actor's Instructions:

Your background:
You are a 52-year-old female called Roya who has come into see the GP because you have been feeling low every day for the past 2 months.

Your behaviour:
You are hunched over and making little eye contact. Speak quietly initially until the candidate has made a good rapport with you. You may begin to cry when you are speaking about the difficult events you have experienced.

Your history of symptoms:
Three months ago you lost your job at a clothing factory. You have found it hard to find another job. You feel like the situation is hopeless and this has extended to other parts of your life. You are beginning to feel as if things are never going to get better. Your mood is worse in the mornings. You no longer enjoy things as you used to. You used to like going to the cinema, reading books and being with your family but recently you haven't enjoyed these activities. Your energy levels are "ok... I guess". Your concentration is really poor at the moment and you are finding it hard to focus in job interviews, follow TV programmes and keep a track of storylines in books. You do not feel guilty and you haven't noticed any changes or slowing down in your body movements.

Although you feel worried and anxious occasionally, this has not changed. You do not have worrying thoughts running through your mind. You do not experience any symptoms of panic or worry that something bad is going to happen. You do not have suicidal thoughts and you would never to do anything to hurt yourself or others. You have clear thoughts for the future including wanting to get help for your low mood and trying to find a job. You do not have psychotic symptoms such as delusions or hallucinations. You have no medical problems and you do not take any medications or have any allergies. You don't drink alcohol for religious reasons and have never tried drugs. You do not smoke.

You are divorced and have two children who are 15 and 18 years old. You are currently unemployed. You have never experienced any previous mental health problems such as depression or elated mood. Your mother suffered with depression before she passed away and had antidepressants that helped her.

Your mental state:
Your appetite is ok and you haven't lost any weight. Your sleep is often disrupted and you are waking up at 4-5am every morning unable to get back to sleep. Your libido hasn't changed and you aren't currently in a relationship.

If asked admit that you feel that you are suffering with depression, you are interested in help with this including antidepressants or therapy.

MILD-MODERATE DEPRESSION STATION OSCE - "Feeling blue"

Task:	Achieved	Not Achieved
Introduces self		
Clarifies who they are speaking to		
Establishes rapport		
Elicits history of symptoms (nature, onset, triggers, timing)		
Establishes timing (most of the day for >2 weeks)		
Establishes core symptoms of depression – (low mood, anhedonia, fatigue)		
Asks about *at least three* biological symptoms of depression (diurnal variation in mood, appetite and weight loss, disturbed sleep, early morning waking, reduced libido)		
Asks about *at least two* other symptoms of depression (guilt, hopelessness, poor concentration or indecisiveness, low Self-confidence, slowing of movement)		
Asks about symptoms of anxiety		
Asks about previous episodes of low or elated mood		
Asks about psychotic symptoms (delusions or hallucinations)		
Asks about self-harm or suicidal thoughts		
Asks about past psychiatric history		
Asks about past medical history		
Asks about medication history and allergies		
Asks about family history (depression, suicide)		
Asks about social history (alcohol, smoking, drugs, employment)		

Asks about personal history (childhood, school, relationships)		
Summarises consultation concisely		
Provides appropriate diagnosis (depression), including the severity (mild-moderate) based on duration and symptoms		
Examiner's Global Mark	/5	
Actor / Helper's Global Mark	/5	
Total Station Mark	/30	

Learning Points

- Depression is an extremely common mental health disorder, affecting 350 million people worldwide and affecting one in five people at some point in their lives. It is likely to present in all healthcare environments.

- A depressive episode can be categorized as mild, moderate or severe depending on the number of symptoms and symptom severity. Symptoms should be present for two weeks or more and every symptom should be present for most of every day. Symptoms can be divided into core, biological and other.

Core symptoms	Biological symptoms	Other symptoms
Low mood Anhedonia Fatigue	Diurnal variations in mood Appetite and weight loss Disturbed sleep including early morning waking Reduced libido	Guilt Hopelessness Poor concentration or indecisiveness Low self-confidence Agitation or slowing of movement

- **Mild depression** (four symptoms)
- **Moderate depression** (five to six symptoms)
- **Severe depression** (seven or more symptoms, with or without psychotic symptoms)

- In the OSCE, a useful way to ask about mood is to ask the patient to rate their mood on a scale of 1 to 10

- It is critical to perform a risk assessment when assessing a patient with low mood. You could always ask to see the patient again in a week's time if you have concerns and want to keep an eye on them.

1.6 "Mirror mirror"

Candidate's Instructions:

You are a foundation year doctor on a community psychiatry placement. You are seeing your own patients this morning. The first patient is a 19-year-old Alexis, who has been referred by their GP.

Take a history. You will be stopped after 7 minutes to summarise your findings and provide a differential diagnosis.

Examiner's Instructions:

A 19-year-old man, Alexis, has been referred by their GP to see a psychiatrist. The GP is concerned because Alexis is disproportionately preoccupied with the fact that his ears are abnormal. As soon as he turned 18 he spent his life savings (£3000) on having ear reshaping (otoplasty) by a plastic surgeon, despite being told that there was no disfigurement by his family, friends, GP and multiple surgeons. He is still unhappy with his ears.

The foundation doctor has been asked to take a history from Alexis in a community psychiatry outpatient clinic.

Please stop the candidate at 7 minutes and ask them to summarise their findings, and provide a differential diagnosis. Prompt the candidate for a differential diagnosis if they do not offer one.

Actor's Instructions:

Background:
You are a 19-year-old male called Alexis who has been referred to a psychiatrist by their GP. For over five years you have felt that your ears are large and stick out like "Mickey Mouse."

Your history of symptoms:
Your concern has grown in intensity over the last year, largely because your hairline is prematurely receding and you think this accentuates the abnormality. You have started carrying a little pocket mirror with you can spend hours gazing into picking out flaws. You feel that your ears are so disfigured and that everyone is talking about them behind your back. You spend hours getting ready in the morning. You have started wearing hats to hide your ears. When you turned 18, you spent your life savings (£3000) on having ear reshaping (otoplasty) by a private plastic surgeon. Tragically, after the surgery you are still unhappy with the shape of your ears.

You were at college doing your A-levels (Photography, Business Studies and Media Studies) but gave up as it was unbearable to have everyone talking behind your back about your ears. You have stopped seeing your friends and going out as you are worried that they were just looking at your "Mickey Mouse" ears.

You smoke 20 cigarettes a day as this calms your nerves. You don't drink regularly but when you do, you drink quite a lot in one go e.g. a bottle of wine and shots on top. You have tried some illicit drugs at college such as 'spice.' You live with your parents and have a 12-year-old brother who you are not close to. You describe a happy childhood, but were bullied at your primary school for being overweight. You have no medical problems, regular medications, no previous contact with mental health services or family history of psychiatric disorders.

Your mental state:
You do not have any psychotic symptoms such as delusions (false fixed beliefs), or hallucinations. You deny any suicidal thoughts and you would never to do anything to hurt yourself or others. You have clear thoughts for the future including trying to find a job. You do not have any other obsessive-compulsive disorder traits such as compulsive hand washing, excessive tidiness, intrusive thoughts or magical thinking. Although your ears make you feel sad at times, you do not have any symptoms of depression such as persistent low mood, tiredness or not enjoying anything. Your appetite and sleep are "normal." You are anxious about your ears and feel uneasy in social situations and in college. But you do not have any other worries and concerns apart from your ears.

Your behaviour:
You are anxious, and when talking about your ears, your hands occasionally move up to cover them. You display partial insight into your concern as, upon questioning you are able to recognise that perhaps your ears aren't as huge as you think, and that other people wouldn't say they stick out. This reassurance lasts only for a few minutes and then you will start saying how big your ears are again. You want help.

If asked, you admit that this could be a mental health problem and that you would like help with it, although you would also like a second opinion from another plastic surgeon.

BODY DYSMORPHIA OSCE - "Mirror Mirror"

Task:	Achieved	Not Achieved
Introduces self		
Clarifies who they are speaking to and gains consent		
Non-judgmental approach		
Establishes history of belief –thoughts, duration, triggers		
Establishes strength of belief – overvalued idea, rather than a fixed delusion		
Establishes strength of preoccupation – money and time spent seeking advise, plastic surgery, mirror gazing, camouflaging, prolonged grooming		
Establishes level of distress caused and impairment of functioning – social isolation, unemployment, poor inter-personal relationships		
Asks about other obsessive-compulsive symptoms (rituals, compulsions, repetitive behaviours)		
Asks about any depressive symptoms (low mood, anhedonia, fatigue)		
Asks about any anxiety symptoms (psychological and biological)		
Asks about any psychotic symptoms – delusions and hallucinations		
Asks about self-harm or suicidal thoughts		
Asks about past psychiatric history		
Asks about past medical history		
Asks about medications and allergies		
Asks about social history (illicit drugs, alcohol, smoking, employment)		

Asks about personal history (childhood, school, relationships)		
Asks about family history of mental illness		
Summarises consultation concisely		
Provides differential diagnosis – Body Dysmorphic Disorder, Delusional Disorder, Depression, OCD		
Examiner's Global Mark	/5	
Actor / Helper's Global Mark	/5	
Total Station Mark	/30	

Learning Points

- Body dysmorphic disorder (BDD) is a variant of hypochondrial disorder. The individual will have a persistent preoccupation with a presumed disfigurement or deformity, for example – crooked nose or ugly hands. The belief is typically an overvalued idea rather than a fixed idea. Those that are fixed ideas (delusions) are classified within delusional disorders (e.g. delusional dysmorphophobia). The preoccupation often results in the person withdrawing from their social life and can cause functional impairment.

- Those suffering with BDD will typically seek help with the perceived disfigurement. However, this is unlikely to help as their concerns as not based in reality. They are at risk from their vulnerability and spending thousands of pounds seeking help or undergoing risky surgical procedures in order to approach their concern.

- In the OSCE, it is important to explore co-morbid psychiatric conditions such as depression, anxiety, social phobia or obsessive-compulsive disorder. Additionally, a dual diagnosis of a drug and or alcohol problem is important to elicit.

- Treatment options include:

Patient Group	Treatment Options
Adults with BDD with mild functional impairment	Course of CBT (including Exposure and Response Prevention) that addresses key features of BDD in individual or group formats.
Adults with BDD with moderate functional impairment	Choice of either a course of an SSRI or more intensive individual CBT (including Exposure and Response Prevention) that addresses key features of BDD
Adults with BDD with severe functional impairment	Combined treatment with an SSRI and CBT (including Exposure and Response Prevention) that addresses key features of BDD.

1.7 "They are controlling us"

Candidate's Instructions:

You are a foundation year doctor in the emergency department. Your next patient is a 21-year-old male called Ahmed who has been brought to the emergency department by the police after being found acting bizarrely in the middle of a busy street.

Please take a history from Ahmed. You will be stopped by the examiner after 7 minutes to summarise and provide a differential diagnosis.

Examiner's Instructions:

The police have brought a 21-year-old male called Ahmed to the emergency department. The foundation year doctor has been asked to take a history from him.

Please stop the candidate at 7 minutes and ask them to summarise and provide a differential diagnosis. Please prompt the candidate to justify the diagnosis if they do not do so, and to explain why.

Actor's Instructions:

Your background:
You are a 21-year-old male called Ahmed. People are watching you and monitoring your every movement through a microchip that has been implanted in your brain. They know where you are going and what you are thinking.

Your mental state:
You are dishevelled, with messy hair and your jumper tied around your head. You are sitting in the corner of the room on the floor muttering and appear to be talking to people who aren't in the room. You don't notice the doctor as they walk in. When they attempt to engage you, you can come and sit on the chair but continue to keep responding to voices. Appear to be actively responding to voices whilst looking at corners of the room (e.g. "yes," "you're right," "ok") and say that they are confirming that we are all being controlled by a central group of elite professionals. You do not know who the voices are but there are two males, and you know they are "safe" and "can be trusted".

Your history of symptoms:
You were in the middle of the busy street trying to tell the public about the people who are watching you, when you were arrested by the police. These voices have been going on for months. They do not talk to you, but talk about you, they describe what you are doing in a running commentary fashion, like a movie. They do not tell you to do things, such as harming others, and you think you would be able to resist it if they did instruct you.

Although you do not think anything is wrong with you mentally, you admit to having had two previous psychiatric admissions. Both were initially under Section 136, followed by Section 3. You were only discharge from your last admission 2 weeks ago and have stopped taking your medication (olanzapine, mirtazapine) and have started smoking cannabis again. You feel that cannabis helps to make things clear such as the messages from the voices. You started smoking cannabis when you were 15 and smoke 4-5 joints every day apart from when you were in hospital.

You do not have any thoughts of hurting yourself or others. You have no medical problems. You do not drink alcohol or take any drugs apart from cannabis. Your brother has paranoid schizophrenia and is currently in hospital. You believe this to be part of the conspiracy. You live at home with your parents. You have never had a proper job and are receiving benefits.

You do not believe that you have a mental health illness and firmly believe that there is a conspiracy involving you and your brother. You do not want help from psychiatric services and do not need medication.

PARANOID SCHIZOPHRENIA OSCE - "THEY ARE CONTROLLING US"

Task:	Achieved	Not Achieved
Introduces self		
Clarifies who they are speaking to and gains consent		
Establishes rapport		
Elicits history of symptoms (nature, onset, triggers, timing)		
Establishes timing of psychotic symptoms (>1month)		
Hallucinations: establishes presence of auditory hallucinations –running commentary and 3rd person auditory hallucinations		
Delusions: establishes presence of persecutory delusions		
Asks about thought insertion, withdrawal, echo and broadcast		
Asks about symptoms of low or high mood		
Asks about suicidal thoughts, risk to self and others		
Asks about past psychiatric history		
Asks about past medical history		
Asks about medication history and allergies		
Asks about family history		
Asks about social history (alcohol, smoking, drugs, employment)		
Asks about personal history (childhood, relationships, school)		
Asks about forensic history		
Summarises consultation concisely		

Provides appropriate diagnosis and suitable differential (delusional disorder, mood disorder with psychosis, organic causes such as epilepsy, drug induced psychosis)		
Non-judgmental approach		
Examiner's Global Mark	/5	
Actor / Helper's Global Mark	/5	
Total Station Mark	/30	

Learning Points

- Paranoid schizophrenia is the most common type of schizophrenia in most parts of the world. Symptoms should be present for most of the time, during a period of 1 month or more.

- **ICD 10 diagnosis guidelines for schizophrenia include:**

One or more of the followings symptoms	Two or more of the following symptoms
Thought echo, insertion, withdrawal, or broadcast Delusions of control or passivity; delusional perception Hallucinatory voices Persistent delusions of other kinds that are culturally inappropriate and completely impossible	Persistent hallucinations in any modality, with fleeting or half-formed delusions or by persistent over-valued ideas Thought disorder Catatonic behaviour Negative symptoms such as marked apathy, paucity of speech, and blunting or incongruity of emotional responses Significant and consistent change in overall quality of personal behaviour

- In the patient with auditory hallucinations, remember to ask about 'command hallucinations' where they are being directly talked to or instructed. Always explore whether the patient would act on these. If they are being told to kill someone, and are unable to resist their hallucinations, this is very high risk!

1.8 "Ka-ching"

Candidate's Instructions:

You are a foundation year doctor working in a GP practice. A young woman of 25, Jessica, is brought in by her partner, who is worried about her. They tell you her behaviour has changed over the past four days – she is unusually energetic, to a concerning extent.

Please perform a full Mental State Examination (MSE). Please do not take a history. You have 5 minutes to do this, after which you will be asked to present the MSE, risk assessment and provide a differential diagnosis.

Examiner's Instructions:

A young woman of 25 called Jessica is brought in by her partner, who is worried about her changing behaviour. The foundation year doctor at the practice has been asked to see her and perform a Mental State Examination (MSE).

Please stop the examination after 5 minutes, and ask the following:

1. Please present the MSE...
2. Please summarise your risk assessment...
3. What do you think the most likely diagnosis is? (Hypomanic episode)

Actor's Instructions:

Background:
You are a 25-year-old called Jessica. Your partner is worried about you. Over the past four days you have been unusually cheerful and elated with poor sleep. You are spending excess money on clothing and meals out. This is out of character and has never happened before. You are still managing to go to work as a graphic designer.

This is a Mental State Examination (MSE) station, so the candidate should not be taking a detailed history. If they ask, you have no past medical or psychiatric history.

Your mental state:

MSE	Description
Appearance and Behaviour	You look well, appropriately-dressed and well-kempt. You are energetic and cheerful. You can engage in the conversation but are over-familiar – e.g. getting very close to the candidate and telling them that they look nice. You use your hands quite a lot.
Speech	Your speech is fast, loud in volume and you are rather verbose.
Mood	You are obviously cheerful, verging on euphoric. When asked how you feel your mood is, be very positive – "great, fantastic, I feel really good". You are sleeping less than usual. Despite this you have a lot of energy and are working late. You are eating less than usual as you don't feel very hungry, one meal a day is enough.
Thought	Thought process – the answers you give are all relevant and can be understood. You give a bit too much information. You don't veer off the topic, or give incomprehensible responses. No-one is interfering with your thoughts. Thought content – You feel full of life. You spent hundreds of pounds on getting an elaborate tattoo of your late grandmother. You are not worried about the financial implications. Your sexual energy has increased lately, even in public places, and you have become very frustrated when your partner refuses to engage. You have been wearing shorter skirts.

	You are not having any thoughts that are delusional in nature. You do not believe you have any special powers or abilities. You do not have any strong religious beliefs or convictions. You do not know why everyone is so worried as you are doing really well at work.
Perception	You are not having any illusions or visual distortions and you are not hearing voices, or seeing anything or anyone that is not there. You are not responding to external stimuli during the review.
Cognition	You know who you are, where you are, and what time it is.
Insight	If asked whether you think your behaviour is unusual, you should minimise it, e.g. "I'm just having a really good week". You do not think you are unwell. You do not think you need medication.
Risk	You do not have any thoughts of hurting yourself or anyone else. You are likely to continue spending money to live life to the fullest despite the financial implications. You do not think you are sexually vulnerable.

P

MSE OSCE - Hypomania

Task:	Achieved	Not Achieved
Introduces self		
Clarifies who they are speaking to and gains consent from patient		
Establishes rapport		
Elicits history of recent behaviours in a concise and fluent manner		
Comments on appearance (height, overweight/underweight, clothing, kempt/unkempt).		
Comments on behaviour (activity levels, fidgety, suspicious)		
Comments on speech (rate/volume/tone)		
Comments on objective mood (low/Euthymic/Elated)		
Comments on affect (reactive/Flat/Blunted)		
Comments on subjective mood (including sleep, appetite, dad, suicidal, Hopeless, Happy, Optimistic).		
Comments specifically about suicidal thoughts and risk		
Comments on thought form (No disorder of thought form)		
Comments on thought content (paranoid thoughts, delusions, grandiosity, financial disinhibition, sexual disinhibition, thought insertion / withdrawal / broadcast)		
Comments on visual hallucinations (What they have seen)		
Comments on auditory hallucinations (E.g. Who the voices are, whether they are 1st, 2nd or 3rd person, what they are saying etc.)		
Comments on cognition (Includes whether patient is orientated in time, place, and person)		
Comments on level of insight "do you think you are unwell?" "Do you think you need medication?"		
Presents MSE concisely and fluently		

Presents a detailed risk assessment (including self-harm, suicide, harming others, sexual vulnerability, financial vulnerability)		
Provides diagnosis and suitable differential (hypomania)		
Examiner's Global Mark	/5	
Actor / Helper's Global Mark	/5	
Total Station Mark	/30	

Learning Points

o   Mental State Examination (MSE) covers a lot of points in a short space of time. It is strictly a point in time snapshot of the patient's mental state and puts your observational and detective skills to the test. It challenges both your skills at eliciting signs and your interpretation of a patient's behaviour and objective appearance. Practice so that it becomes second nature and you don't miss any major areas under pressure. As with all clinical examinations, find a structure that works for you and stick with it. Do not forget a risk assessment.

o   Hypomania is characterized by elevated mood for 4 days or more. It is important to differentiate it from from mania; the lack of psychotic features and the maintained social functioning are more suggestive of hypomania.

o   When thinking about further investigations for any psychiatric patient, always start by ruling out organic causes. These may include blood tests (particularly thyroid function and electrolyte imbalances such as hypercalcaemia), neuroimaging (CT or MRI), particularly if a first presentation, and a urine drug screen

1.9 "Come fly with me"

Candidate Instructions

You are a foundation year doctor working in a GP Surgery. Today you are seeing a 45-year-old man called Nathan, who would like some pills for his fear of flying.

Please take a history. At 7 minutes you will be asked to summarise your findings and provide an initial management plan.

Examiner Instructions

A 45-year-old man called Nathan has attended his GP surgery. He has developed a fear of flying which is impacting on his ability to function in his new job. He would like some pills to help cope with this. The foundation doctor at the practice has been asked to take a history.

Please stop the candidate after 7 minutes and ask them to summarise their findings and provide an initial management plan.

Actors Instructions

Background:
You are a 45-year-old man called Nathan. You visited your GP as you have developed a severe phobia of flying which is impacting on your ability to do your new job. You ideally want a prescription for some medication to "cure" this.

Your behaviour:
You are embarrassed about your fear of flying at your age. You are quite pushy with the doctor to obtain some pills to "cure" this. During the interview you are calm and relaxed, but when you discuss the incident of the flight and the panic attack, you become anxious and your speech becomes louder and faster.

History of symptoms:
You have always found flying quite unpleasant and tended to avoid it if possible. However, you were able to tolerate short flights if absolutely necessary. Six months ago you took a flight to Italy with business and there was severe turbulence. Whilst on the plane you had a panic attack and were taken to hospital once it landed. You felt sweaty, your heart was racing, you felt nauseous and the tips of your fingers were tingling. Thankfully all the tests at the hospital were normal. You tried to fly back from Italy but were unable to board the plane and nearly had another panic attack at the gate. You were forced to take the high-speed train home. This was very embarrassing as you had to split up from your work colleagues. Since then you have had a severe phobia of the experience of flying.

Your new job is a big promotion and you are being asked to fly abroad for business meetings much more often. So far you have managed to make up excuses to avoid being posted on most of the foreign projects. On a few occasions this was unavoidable and you bought some Diazepam over the internet. You are worried because you know they can be addictive, and want to speak to the GP about alternative cures. Soon, there is a meeting being held in the USA which you are integral to. You are becoming increasingly anxious at just the thought of flying. When your mind isn't thinking about flying you are a fairly relaxed person – before the flight incident, you had never had a panic attack. Your anxieties now seem very focused on flying, thoughts of flying or even just being near airports. Your drive home used to take you right past Heathrow airport and now you take a different route.

You fully understand that the phobia is irrational and that flying is the safest form of transport, but this does nothing to counteract the sense of panic. You are very worried about the impact this will have on your new job and fear you could even be made redundant. You have found this quite troubling, but you have not felt particularly depressed. You have not felt low or had any thoughts of self-harm or suicide. You are still sleeping and eating well and continue to enjoy playing golf and spending time with your children. You are simply eager to try and resolve, or "cure", this fear.

You have no past psychiatric history. You have no history of obsessive thoughts, or compulsive behaviours. You have no past medical history and take no medications. You have no allergies. You live with your partner in a 3 bed house and have no children. You are a non-smoker and your drink around 3 pints of beer per week. You have no history of recreational drug use. Your mother had a phobia of heights. You have always been a high achiever, and describe a happy childhood.

MSE Phobia OSCE– "Come Fly with Me"

Task:	Achieved	Not Achieved
Introduces self		
Clarifies who they are speaking to and gains consent		
Elicits nature of phobia (nature, onset, triggers, timing, exacerbating factors)		
Elicits biological symptoms of anxiety (sweating, palpitations, parasthesiae)		
Elicits that anxiety is provoked specifically by flying		
Elicits avoidance behaviours (avoids flying, avoids driving near airport)		
Elicits that patient understands fear is irrational		
Elicits impact that phobia is having on patient's life and functioning (ability to do job)		
Asks about obsessive/compulsive symptoms (E.g. obsessive thoughts about cleanliness/contamination. Checking and re-checking behaviours, ritualistic behaviours etc.)		
Elicits that patient has been self-medicating with diazepam)		
Asks about mood / depressive symptoms (E.g. sleep / appetite / concentration / interests)		
Asks about self-harm or suicidal thoughts		
Asks about past psychiatric history		
Asks about past medical history		
Asks about medication history and allergies		
Asks bout family history		
Asks about social history (alcohol, smoking, drugs, employment)		
Asks about personal history (childhood, relationships, school)		
Summarises consultation concisely		

Provides an appropriate initial management plan – must include some form of psychological therapy. Explains that benzodiazepines are useful in short term but in long term can cause dependence. (E.g. CBT/systematic desensitisation, or simply to refer to a psychologist)		
Examiner's Global Mark	/5	
Actor / Helper's Global Mark	/5	
Total Station Mark	/30	

Learning Points

- Specific phobia is the most common psychiatric disorder and occurs in 9.4% to 12.5% of the general population [1].

- It is important to ask about the phobia's impact on an individual's ability to function and to clarify that it is not better accounted for by other conditions such as panic disorder or OCD.

- Panic disorder is characterised by a history of multiple severe panic attacks. In panic disorder, the attacks are not restricted to any situation or set of circumstances and are therefore unpredictable.

  The essential feature of Obsessive Compulsive Disorder (OCD) is the presence of obsessive thoughts and compulsive acts. In OCD, the obsessions tend to be more pervasive, rather than restricted to one specific fear. Compulsive acts are typically ritualised and repeated again and again, and this behaviour is uncommon in specific phobia.

- Psychological therapy is the mainstay of treatment. Most phobias respond to gradual exposure, but there are high dropout rates. The evidence base for medication is limited. Benzodiazepines are effective in managing anxiety in the short term, but have a high risk of leading to dependence and may lead to even worse rebound anxiety when they are stopped.

1.10 - "I only want to speak to the consultant"

Candidate instructions

You are a foundation year doctor working on a secure psychiatric ward, you have been asked by the nursing staff to come and speak with Rafael. He is the son of one of your patients and you have been warned that he appears angry.

Please meet with Rafael to explore his concerns. You have 8 minutes.

Examiner instructions

The foundation year doctor working on a secure psychiatric ward has been asked to speak to the son of one of the patients, Rafael, who is angry. The candidate should meet with Rafael and speak with him in a way that de escalates his anger, remains non-confrontational but also tries to address his concerns and provide some reassurance.

The candidate should remain calm in the face of threats by the relative and should not make derogatory comments about colleagues in order to win the relatives favour.

Pay close attention of the candidate's body language and voice, they should aim to lower the tone and volume of their voice and appear attentive to the angry relative.

Actor Instructions

Background
You are 37-year-old man called Rafael. Your elderly father has a long standing history of bipolar disorder and has recently been detained under Section 3 of the Mental Health Act (1983). You have come to the hospital today and speak with the consultant as you are not happy with some of things you have witnessed on the ward.

Incident
Yesterday when you were on the ward you could see a group of nurses sat in the office chatting. And when your father knocked on the door he was ignored for several minutes. When somebody did answer the door, your father told the nurse that he wanted to go for a cigarette, but was told he would have to come back later because it was 'handover', this left your father quite agitated and distressed, which made you very angry.

You think it's very rude that the nurses all sit in the office having a chat and ignoring the patients. In your mind, the nurses should be trying to calm the patients down rather than distressing them even further. Additionally, you noticed that the linen cupboard was very dirty and that your father's bedding hasn't been changed for several days. You have taken pictures to prove this.

You are thinking about suing the trust for negligence or at least going to the press with the photos and telling them about this incident.

Behaviour
When you learn that you have to speak to the trainee doctor you start to get increasingly irritated and pace up and down. You are initially reluctant to sit down and speak to the trainee doctor. You feel very annoyed that you have to talk to a trainee that is younger than you are, who may not be able to make any useful decisions. You doubt they know much about your father. You think it is

unacceptable that the consultant is not on the ward to hear your concerns and that your father's care has been left in the hands of a trainee doctor. You are feeling very upset and quite angry, a confrontational or defensive approach from the doctor is likely to heighten your anxiety and increase the volume of your voice.

If you feel that the candidate has taken you seriously and listened to your concerns, you start to feel calmer and less worried about your father.

OSCE Station – "I only want to speak to the consultant'

Task:	Achieved	Not Achieved
Introduces self		
Clarifies who they are speaking to and gains consent		
Establishes rapport		
Listens attentively to patients concerns		
Invites the relative to sit down to avoid confrontation		
Apologises early for the consultant's absence and thanks the patient for speaking with them		
Explains their role within the ward and offers to be of help or gives patient option of coming back to speak to consultant at another time		
Makes empathetic statements "it must be very difficult to see a relative in hospital"		
Modifies speech and body language to de-escalate confrontation		
Appears to be non-defensive regarding the relatives complaint "I completely understand why that would upset you", "I'm very sorry your father had that experience"		
Explains the importance of the nursing handover process including passing on important information		
Offers to speak with the nurse about the incident		
Does not implicate nursing staff or collude with patient		
Explain that relatives views and opinions are considered very important to the team and any complaints are taken very seriously		
Explains there is a formal complaints procedure that the relative can follow if they wish, offers telephone number or leaflet for Patient Advice Liaison Service (PALS)		
Does not become flustered after threat of suing or talking to the press and explains taking legal action is within their rights.		
Explains that it is not possible to use images taken on their phone with people in without their consent		

Reassure relative that you will relay the information to the consultant as soon as possible		
Remains calm		
Non-judgemental approach		
Examiner's Global Mark	/5	
Actor / Helper's Global Mark	/5	
Total Station Mark	/30	

Learning points:

- When dealing with an angry patient or relative always try and encourage them to sit down, having a conversation standing up can appear confrontational.

- In communication terms anger has a purpose - to gain the listener's attention. In this case, it is wise for the doctor to give the patient their full attention.

- To increase the sense of empathy lower the tone and volume a bit of your voice and look extra attentive with eye contact at the patient/relative. This makes you sound much more convincing! The NHS has a Zero Tolerance policy for physical aggression from patients or relatives, this should be reported immediately to security team immediately if you feel your safety is being compromised.

1.11 "The self harmer"

Candidate's Instructions:

A 25-year-old lady called Phoebe attends the emergency department (ED) following an episode of deliberate self-harm (DSH).

She has been medically cleared by the ED registrar who informs you that she has a known history of Emotionally unstable personality disorder (EUPD).

You are the foundation doctor on the liaison psychiatry team and have been asked by your registrar to take a history from the patient, with a view to forming a differential diagnosis and management plan.

You have seven minutes to take the history followed by one minute of questions.

Examiner's Instructions:

A 25-year-old lady called Phoebe attends the emergency department following an episode of deliberate self-harm. She has been medically cleared by the emergency department registrar.

The foundation doctor on the liaison psychiatry team has been asked to take a detailed history from the patient with a view to forming a differential diagnosis and initial management plan.

Pay particular attention to the candidate's interaction with this young lady who is prone to becoming irritable and defensive. If the candidate fails to establish a good rapport, the actor may threaten to end the discussion.

At 7 minutes, please ask the candidate to summarise the case, and then ask the following two questions:

1. What differential diagnoses would you consider for this patient?

2. What would you like to include in your initial management plan?

Actor's Instructions:

Background

You are a 25-year-old lady called Phoebe who has self-presented to the emergency department after deliberately cutting parts of your body (upper arms, upper legs and stomach). You have been seen by the emergency department registrar who felt that no stitches or other medical interventions were required.

Your behaviour

You have attended the emergency department voluntarily to have your cuts assessed as you thought they might need stitches. However, once you were informed this wasn't necessary, you wanted to go home immediately and are annoyed that you now have to wait to see a psychiatry doctor. You are prone to becoming irritable and angry when you feel people aren't listening to you properly, or don't truly care about your needs. If the candidate doesn't act sensitively towards you, you threaten to walk out of the consultation. At first you are guarded with your information, giving only one word answers, but if the candidate gains your trust you reveal the more intimate parts of your life story.

Your history of symptoms

You have been self-harming since the age of 12. This started as superficial cuts to your wrists using razors. You then started to cut other parts of your body such as the tops of your legs, arms, and neck, but you like to keep this hidden so you wear long sleeved clothes and a scarf. Cutting gives you a feeling of release of tension. You have carried out other forms of self-harm such as swallowing bleach and batteries. You have taken several overdoses in the past, of about 10 paracetamol tablets on each occasion with a bottle of vodka. One of the overdoses followed a break-up with your ex-boyfriend and you were admitted to a psychiatric unit.

You grew up with your mother and father. However, your father raped you repeatedly between the ages of 5 and 10. The abuse stopped because your father committed suicide. You tried to tell your mum what was happening on more than one occasion but she didn't believe you. You have a volatile relationship with your mum and you are convinced that she doesn't truly love you.

You didn't enjoy school. and left when you were 16. You were suspended several times due to acts of unprovoked aggression and violence towards school teachers, and were nearly expelled twice for throwing chairs at other students. Your friendships never lasted long and there was a period when you were verbally bullied. Your school reports also said that you were prone to lying, for example telling everyone that you were rich and that your dad was a famous actor who had been killed in a car crash. You now work at call centre but your boss is threatening to sack you as you have had frequent days off work for stress.

You find it difficult to trust people, particularly men. You are in a relationship with a female at the moment (although you don't label yourself as gay). It's a "rocky" relationship and you have frequent arguments and break-ups. You are convinced that she will leave you and think she is probably having an affair.

There are times in your life when you feel sad and empty. These tend to be triggered by something that reminds you of the rapes, such as a particular song that you may hear on the radio. During these times you carry out self-harm.

You have not experienced any unusual symptoms such as hearing voices or seeing things that other people can't see. You don't have any preoccupation with religion or ideas that your thoughts are being tampered with. You are not currently feeling suicidal and did not intend to end of your life with this current episode of self-harm.

You have no medical conditions and are not on any regular medications. You don't have any allergies. You drink a couple of bottles of wine and some "shots" at the weekend when out with your friends. You occasionally use ecstasy.

Markscheme – "The Self-harmer"

Task:	Achieved	Not Achieved
Introduces self and explains purpose of discussion		
Clarifies to whom they are speaking and gains consent		
Asks about the presenting complaint of self-harm to determine if it was a suicide attempt		
Asks about previous self-harm and suicidal ideation		
Attempts to identify triggers for the episodes of crisis		
Enquires about relationships (childhood, family, partners) and their stability		
Asks about education (schooling) and employment		
Asks about impulsivity and unpredictability		
Asks about bouts of anger/outbursts of temper		
Asks about low mood/feelings of emptiness		
Excludes symptoms of psychosis (hallucinations/delusions)		
Asks about past medical and psychiatric history		
Asks about family history (mental health and suicide)		
Asks about illicit drug use / alcohol misuse		
Performs a risk assessment		
Maintains a calm and non-judgemental approach		
Gains the patient's trust (as evidenced by the patient revealing her full story)		
Avoids "down-playing" the current crisis which was not an actual suicide attempt		
Summarises consultation and offers a differential diagnosis		

Explains a basic management plan (e.g. referral to community mental health services, crisis plan, psychotherapy)		
	/20	
Examiner's Global Mark	/5	
Actor / Helper's Global Mark	/5	
Total Station Mark	/30	

Learning points

- The key to eliciting a meaningful history in a patient with EUPD is to establish a rapport and gain their trust.

- Don't be tempted to "down-play" their suicide risk on the basis that they have made repeated threats. One in ten people will EUPD will die from suicide

- Psychotherapy (such as teaching tools to deal with difficult emotions) is one of the most effective forms of treatment but is not a short-term solution and a patient may require twice-weekly sessions for one to two years.

- You may find it helpful to offer the patient a questionnaire. A diagnosis can usually be made if the patient answers "yes" to five or more of the following questions: 3

  - Do you have a fear of being left alone?

  - Do you have intense and unstable relationships?

  - Do you ever feel you don't have a strong sense of your own self?

• Do you engage in impulsive activities in two areas that are potentially damaging, such as unsafe sex, drug abuse or reckless spending?

• Have you made repeated suicide threats or attempts in your past and engaged in self-harming?

• Do you have severe mood swings, such as feeling intensely depressed, anxious or irritable, which last from a few hours to a few days?

• Do you have long-term feelings of emptiness and loneliness?

• Do you often find it difficult to control your anger?

• When you find yourself in stressful situations, do you feel like you're disconnected from the world or from your own body?

1.12 "Out of sorts"

Candidate's Instructions:

A 23-year-old lady called Ling has presented to the emergency department accompanied with her friend, who is concerned that she has been 'out of sorts'.

You are a foundation doctor working in the emergency department and have been asked by your consultant to take a brief history and Mental state examination (MSE) from the patient.

You have 6 minutes to take your history after which you will be asked to summarise the MSE and provide an initial management plan.

Examiner's Instructions:

A 23-year-old lady called Ling has come into the emergency department She is 6 weeks postpartum. Her friend was concerned with her recent behaviour so has brought her in for assessment. Currently Ling looks anxious and seems to acting oddly and responding to voices.

The foundation doctor in the emergency department has been asked to take a brief history and present the Mental State Examination (MSE).

At 6 minutes stop the candidate and ask them to summarise the MSE, and what they would include in their initial management plan.

Actor's Instructions:

Background
You are a 23-year-old lady called Ling. Your friend has brought you into the hospital today; you do not understand why he is concerned. You gave birth 6 weeks ago to your first child and are worried that your baby will be taken away from you.

Your Mental State
Your appearance is unkempt and you have a closed defensive posture. Your behaviour is irritable. Your speech is slow and disjointed; you sometimes find it difficult to recall thoughts. You feel low in mood and hopeless as a mother. You hear voices that only you can hear telling you that you are a terrible mother. You randomly shout in response saying "I'm not a bad mother, I'm trying my best!". The voices sometimes command you to end it all and you find it difficult to resist this temptation. You are not experiencing any visual or tactile hallucinations. You do not believe there is anything wrong with you. You refuse any medication or treatment and accuse the doctor of working with social services to take your son away.

Your history of symptoms
Your friend is concerned about your recent behaviour as he found you locked in your bathroom with your child. The voices have told you that you are unfit to be a mother and that social services are monitoring you through radio waves. You have not been able to sleep or eat for weeks but are full of energy.

You had a planned pregnancy, however during the pregnancy you split from your partner and have not heard from him since. Towards the end of the pregnancy you were admitted to hospital with bleeding and had an emergency caesarean section at 30 weeks, which was a very traumatic experience. You have not bonded with your baby as he was kept in hospital due to medical complications and came home 2 weeks ago. Since he has come home you have struggled to take care of him alone and have barely slept. The nurses say that he is underweight. You have tried to breastfeed but he fusses so much that you have given up trying to feed him more than once a day.

You have no personal history of mental illness. You were adopted so do not know if you have a family history of psychiatric illness. You have no other significant medical history, regular medications or drug allergies.

You have not harmed yourself yet, but you have been tempted to end it all like the voices tell you to. You have not made any clear plans yet. You feel like there is nothing that will prevent you from trying to commit suicide and say "everyone will be better off without me." The voices have not told you to harm your baby and you do not have the temptation to do so.

You used to drink ½ a bottle of wine a day but stopped when you found out you were pregnant. You used to work in a shop. You have no support at home apart from a friend who lives with you.

Markscheme – postpartum

Task:	Achieved	Not Achieved
Introduces the conversation and confirms the patient's identity		
Elicits history from patient in a concise manner		
Asks about presenting complaint		
Asks about depressive symptoms – low mood, energy levels and sleep disturbances (early morning wakening)		
Asks about psychotic symptoms - delusions, auditory, visual and tactile hallucinations		
Asks about preconception period – young, first time mothers, support system, planned or unplanned pregnancy		
Asks about antenatal period – medical problems, social issues, support		
Asks about the birth – traumatic delivery, medical intervention, support		
Asks about postnatal period – support, bonding, mood, coping		
Asks specifically about self harm and suicidal ideation – thoughts of suicide, plans, final acts (writing a will, leaving a note, ensuring you wouldn't be found)		
Asks about risk of harm to child – emotional, physical, sexual abuse and neglect		
Asks about protective factors to prevent suicide – family support, carers, partners		
Asks about past medical history		

Asks about past psychiatric history		
Asks about family history		
Asks drug and alcohol history		
Assesses insight – ability to recognize there is a problem and accept treatment		
Presents the Mental State Examination fluently		
Structured management plan: conservative therapies – CBT, admission to mother-baby unit, paediatric team involvement, safeguarding, social services, community psychiatry nurses, midwife input. Medical management – anti-psychotics, anti-depressants, ECT for persistent symptoms		
Examiner's Global Mark	/5	
Actor / Helper's Global Mark	/5	
Total Station Mark	/30	

Learning Points

- Differentiate between baby blues, postpartum depression and postpartum psychosis. Post partum depression can occur up to 1 year postpartum, symptoms of low mood, reduced energy and anhedonia. This requires treatment unlike baby blues, which lasts a few days to a week. Postpartum psychosis usually presents in the first 2 weeks postpartum with florid psychotic features. These are extremely high risk and vulnerable patients, and are often all admitted to Mother & Baby Units.
- Determine the timeline of events from pre-conception through to the post partum period to find risk factors for post partum psychosis. These include unsupported first time mothers, antenatal medical problems, traumatic delivery, prematurity and difficulties during the post partum period.

- Be as specific as you can with regards to suicidal risk, you need to assess if the patient is likely to harm themselves or their child. Ascertain if they have made a plan or committed any final acts such as writing a will.

1.13 "Nasty neighbours"

Candidate's Instructions:

A 27-year-old man called Kryz has been brought into the emergency department by the police on Section 136. He was found agitated in the city centre. Police say that he has been talking 'nonsense' and was found climbing onto private property.

You are a foundation doctor in the emergency department and have been asked to perform a Mental State Examination (MSE). You do not need to take a detailed history of the symptoms.

You will be stopped after 5 minutes to summarise the findings of your MSE, provide a differential diagnosis and management plan.

Examiner's Instructions:

The candidate has been asked to complete a Mental State Examination (MSE) on Kryz, a 27-year-old male brought into the emergency department by police on Section 136. He was found agitated in the city centre, talking 'nonsense' and was found climbing onto private property

The candidate should focus on performing the MSE rather than take a history.

Please stop the candidate after 5 minutes and ask them to summarise the MSE, provide a differential diagnosis and management plan.

Please look out for the following phrases when the candidate is presenting the MSE:

MSE component	Description
Appearance and behaviour	Anxious, casually dressed, dirty clothes, poor eye contact, fidgety, irritated, difficulty concentrating
Speech	Pressure of speech, normal form and content
Mood and affect	Stressed, nervous, scared, anxious, paranoid, irritable. Mood is not low or elated
Thought	Secondary delusion of a persecutory nature and normal thought form
Perception	Third person auditory hallucinations, some visual illusions e.g. cameras
Cognition	Poor concentration, orientated
Insight	No insight
Risk	Medium risk to himself – not eating, poor sleep, may get hurt whilst 'removing cameras' around the city. High risk to neighbours – has had thoughts of attacking neighbours for the good of society, only protective factor is that the police won't believe him

Actor's Instructions:

Background:
You are Mark, a 27-year-old man who has been taken into the emergency department by the police on Section 136 because you were found to be agitated in the city centre.

Overall impression:
You are overtly anxious, suspicious and paranoid about everyone around you. You are angry at the staff, but also scared of them, because they are all 'part of it'. You have been under a lot of stress lately; you weren't causing trouble in the city you were just trying to help. You can be irritable, especially if you don't think the candidate is empathetic. You are dressed in dirty walking gear and trainers and have a large bag with you full of things you might need 'just in case'. You talk quickly, your eye contact is poor and your legs are constantly fidgeting because you are nervous. You have difficulty concentrating on the conversation.

Thoughts and beliefs:
On further questioning you tell the doctor that your stress is because of the difficulties you are having with your neighbours. It all started with a petty argument about the bins and escalated from there. Since then they seem to have something against you and have been making your life hell.

You believe that they are putting cameras everywhere in your house and around the city disguised in ordinary objects to keep an eye on you. You have had to throw away your TV, radio and lots of other items because of this. Today, you were trying to destroy some of these cameras hidden around the city. They are very well hidden and even though you think you can see a camera you can never actually find one. You have also covered your ceiling with tin foil to protect you against the radiation that they are sending down onto your flat. You have had thoughts about attacking your neighbours in order to protect society but you don't think the police would believe you.

You sometimes feel like your thoughts become muddled, and that is probably due to the radiation. However, you do not think that anyone is putting thoughts into your head, blocking or taking your thoughts.

Perceptions:
You can hear your neighbours talking about you, these voices are not in your head, they are clear and they are coming though the walls or down the pipes. There are 2 voices, one male and one female, but they aren't the real voices of your neighbours, that's because they use a disguise. They often say bad things about you, and talk about their next plan. The voices don't talk directly to you, they don't command you to do things and they don't comment on what you are doing.

Mood and affect:
You have been understandably extremely anxious, and you constantly have to be prepared which is very stressful. Your sleep is erratic and your appetite is poor, due to all the stress the neighbours are causing you. You haven't left the house lately because you think they are waiting for you to do so, in order for them to install more cameras. You couldn't possibly be that predictable, which means you've had to make excuses not to go to work at the local supermarket. Despite all this you don't feel down, depressed or suicidal in any way.

Cognition:
You have not had any problems with your memory, you are not confused and you are orientated to time, place and person. You are annoyed that the doctor would ask you about these things 'I'm not stupid'.

Insight:

You have no insight into your mental state. You have absolutely no doubt that this is all true, but you don't know why everyone is so against you. You think that some of the staff at the hospital could be 'in on it' too so you are keen to get out as soon as possible. You try and convince the doctor to let you go so you can get to safety. You are not willing to stay and not willing to receive treatment because there isn't anything wrong with you.

MSE STATION – Nasty neighbours

Task:	Achieved	Not Achieved
Introduces self		
Confirms patient identity and gains consent		
Asks about mood		
Asks about suicidal ideation and plans		
Asks about thought disorder (insertion, broadcasting and removal)		
Asks about delusional thought content (control, grandiose, reference, persecutory)		
Elicits persecutory delusion and confirms absolute certainty		
Elicits risk to self and others		
Asks about hallucinations (visual, tactile, olfactory, auditory, gustatory)		
Elicits characteristics/content of the hallucinations		
Differentiates if the voices are 2nd or 3rd person		
Assesses cognition (orientation, attention/concentration, recalling events)		
Asks about insight		
Summarises the MSE fluently		
Comments on positive findings (see examiner's instructions)		
Identifies correct delusions and hallucinations		
Gives appropriate diagnosis of paranoid schizophrenia		
Provides appropriate differential diagnosis		
Suggests appropriate management plan (e.g referral to liaison psychiatry team for assessment/admission or high intensity community support, medication)		
Develops rapport and shows empathy		
Examiner's Global Mark	/5	
Actor / Helper's Global Mark	/5	
Total Station Mark	/30	

Learning Points

- It is vital to assess suicide risk on every patient you see with psychiatric symptoms, even if this isn't the focus of the station. If you're unsure of their risk always involve a senior.

- The first rank symptoms of schizophrenia were devised by German psychiatrist Kurt Schneider are a collection of symptoms, commonly seen in, but not pathognomonic of patients with schizophrenia. Their presence can therefore aid with diagnosis.

  They can be broadly categorised into four types which include:

  1. Auditory Hallucinations: particularly third person, commentary or thought echo
  2. Thought disorder: thought broadcasting, insertion or withdrawal
  3. Delusions of control: Passivity phenomena including passivity of impulse, volitions or affect. Somatic passivity may also occur.
  4. Delusional perception: A delusionary belief where a patient attributes meaning or a message to an everyday perception

Illusions are not true hallucinations. For example, this patient thinking there are cameras in/on ordinary objects is an illusion secondary to the delusion. If this was a 'true' visual hallucination, he would be able to see the cameras

1.14 "Anxious annie"

Candidate's Instructions:

You are a foundation doctor in a suburban GP practice where Annie, a 32-year-old lady has come to see you. You can see from the GP records that she has not seen a GP in quite a few years and has no significant past medical history. She did not attend her scheduled GP appointment last week due to 'anxiety'.

You have 7 minutes to take a focused history from this patient and make a primary diagnosis.

Examiner's Instructions:

The candidate is a foundation doctor working in a suburban GP surgery. They have been asked to take a history from Anne, a 32-year-old lady who has come to see her GP due to increasing anxiety and fear of leaving the house.

Pay particular attention to the candidate's communication skills and their ability to put an anxious patient at ease. You also need to assess their awareness of anxiety disorders and ability to take a focused history.

Please stop the candidate after 7 minutes and ask them to summarise their findings and give a diagnosis.

Actor's Instructions:

Background
You are a 32-year-old housewife called Annie with 2 young children of 3 and 5 years old. You have come to see the GP because your eldest daughter has recently started school and you haven't been able to take her there yourself because it makes you feel too anxious.

You think it all started 3 weeks ago you when you were dropping your daughter off at school and you suddenly became really unwell. During this episode you felt dizzy, sweaty, couldn't breathe properly and had pain in your chest. You thought you were having a heart attack and it felt like you were dying. Luckily, a passer-by called an ambulance and the paramedics arrived quickly. You were only in hospital for a few hours before the doctors discharged you with the diagnosis of a panic attack, but you don't think this can be true because your symptoms were real. This all happened near the school entrance with lots of parents around and you felt humiliated by the experience. You're embarrassed to talk about it, and are terrified that if you leave the house it will happen again, and potentially cause serious harm to your health. A few months ago you had 2 similar episodes in the supermarket, but these weren't as severe and resolved after 4 to 5 minutes.

Since the event you have been unable to take your daughter to school due to feeling anxious when you get near the front door. This makes you think you're are a bad mother and you feel extremely guilty. You haven't left the house since the episode and, upon reflection, you realise you have hardly left the house in the last 6 months. You often make excuses to avoid social occasions, do your shopping online and rarely take your children out. However, you think this is because you have 2 young children who take up all your time and they prefer playing in the garden rather than the park.

You have always been quite a shy person and never liked going to events with crowds or big social occasions. Nevertheless, you did used to enjoy meeting up with your close friends and family and taking your children to the local swimming pool but you haven't done this for a few months now. You spend your days playing games with the children in the house. You often can't get to sleep because you are worried about these attacks. You do sometimes feel hopeless and find yourself crying for no reason, but you have never self harmed or thought about suicide. You don't drink alcohol or take drugs, and have no past medical history or drug allergies. You smoke 10 to 20 cigarettes a day, and have noticed that you are smoking more than usual at the moment. You haven't had any problems with concentration and your energy levels and appetite have been normal. As a child you had a normal upbringing and never had any problems at school.

Your husband is very supportive and encouraged you to see the doctor because he thinks you are on edge all the time and have trouble relaxing. He took the day off work to come with you today because you were scared to leave the house alone.

Behaviour
You have very poor eye contact, spending most of the consultation looking down into your lap and are very shy. You are very fidgety, sat on the edge of the chair constantly rubbing your hands together or fiddling with the edge of your clothing.

Questions and actions
You do not volunteer information unless directly asked, answer minimally. You are extremely anxious and need lots of reassurance, but you become more open if you feel the doctor has put you at ease.

HISTORY TAKING OSCE STATION- Anxious Anne

Task:	Achieved	Not Achieved
Introduces self		
Clarifies who they are speaking to and gains consent		
Asks about precipitating events/triggers		
Elicits at least 2 psychological symptoms (fatigue, sleep pattern, irritability, worry, concentration, guilt, feeling of doom)		
Elicits at least 2 somatic symptoms (sweating, palpitations, butterflies, restlessness, hyperventilation, palpitations)		
Impact on daily living and social function		
Asks about symptoms that differentiate anxiety disorders (obsessions, compulsions, repetitive thoughts, avoiding public places, previous trauma)		
Asks about symptoms of depression (low mood, anhedonia, fatigue, lack of concentration)		
Elicits details of premorbid personality – (e.g before these attacks did she have any problems leaving the house		
Past psychiatric history		
Past medical history and medication history		
Briefly asks about birth/development/school		
Elicits substance use (alcohol, smoking, drugs)		
Assess risk of suicide/self harm		
Summarises fluently		
Provides correct diagnosis (agoraphobia) and suitable differential (panic disorder, social phobia, generalised anxiety disorder)		
Appropriate initial management and follow up offered		
Builds rapport with patient		
Empathetic		
Reassures patient		
Examiner's Global Mark	/5	
Actor / Helper's Global Mark	/5	
Total Station Mark	/30	

Learning Points

- Agoraphobia is a fear of crowds/open spaces and the patient usually feels safer at home. Agoraphobia is distinguished from general anxiety disorder by predominantly phobic symptoms rather than constant worry/anxiety.

- 75% of patients with agoraphobia are women between late teens and mid 30's.

- First line treatment includes reassurance, providing diagnosis and education. If symptoms fail to improve then refer for psycho-educational groups or individual guided self help before considering step 3. However, if a patient has marked functional impairment then one can skip to step 3 (individual high intensity psychological intervention and/or medication).

1.15 "Not another medication doc"

Candidate's Instructions:

You have been asked to speak to a 43-year-old male called Liam diagnosed with paranoid schizophrenia 5 years ago. He has already been trialled on 2 different anti-psychotics with little effect. Your consultant reviewed him earlier in the psychiatry outpatient clinic and has advised starting clozapine.

Your colleague has already performed a physical examination, ECG and bloods all of which were normal. Liam has no past medical history and no known drug allergies.

You are the foundation doctor on your psychiatry placement and your consultant has asked you to discuss clozapine treatment with this patient. You have 8 minutes.

Examiner's Instructions:

The candidate has been asked to speak to a 43-year-old male called Liam diagnosed with paranoid schizophrenia 5 years ago. He has already been trialled on 2 different anti-psychotics with little effect. His consultant reviewed him earlier in the psychiatry outpatient clinic and has advised starting clozapine.

Their colleague has already performed a physical examination, ECG and bloods all of which were normal. Liam has no past medical history and no known drug allergies.

The candidate has been asked to counsel this patient regarding their clozapine treatment. They have 8 minutes.

Actor's Instructions:

Background
You are a 43-year-old male called Liam who was diagnosed with paranoid schizophrenia 5 years ago. You have tried 2 different anti-psychotic medications (olanzapine, aripiprazole) and neither seemed to 'make any difference' even at maximal doses. Your symptoms have worsened recently and you came to see the consultant in clinic today because you have been hearing voices more frequently. The consultant recommended that you should try a new 'atypical' anti-psychotic. You have been informed that one of the foundation doctors will need to discuss the medication with you, but you don't know why.

You have been hearing voices in your head for many years. You can hear multiple voices talking to each other, saying horrible things about you and laughing at you. Most of the time you find ways to ignore them but sometimes they don't stop and recently you have damaged a car due to frustration and this got you into trouble with the police. They make you feel worthless and guilty making it difficult for you to be happy in life. You have never injured yourself or thought about committing suicide.

You have no past medical history, have never been admitted to hospital, and have no known drug allergies. There is no family history of medical problems.

Your behaviour
You are quiet and reserved. Poor eye contact throughout and mildly distracted. You are not very interested in what the doctor has to say and you're not sure why you need to try another tablet. You have limited insight into your condition and don't think that another tablet will help you.

Questions and actions

If asked 'do you understand?' just nod in agreement. Although, on further questioning it is quite apparent you don't understand and are in need of further clarification. You are quite reluctant to try a new medication, especially one with lots of side effects, but at the end of the consultation you agree to try the medication.

MEDICATION COUNSELING STATION OSCE - Clozapine

Task:	Achieved	Not Achieved
Introduces self		
Clarifies who they are speaking to and gains consent		
Explains reason for consultation		
Explains rationale behind starting clozapine (e.g for schizophrenia when 2 other anti-psychotics have been ineffective)		
Briefly explains mechanism of action ("works by blocking overactive brain messengers and balancing hormone levels in the brain")		
Explains can take few weeks to have full effect		
Explains risk of low white cell count, agranulocytosis		
Explains it can interfere with the heart causing palpitations and cardiomyopathy/myocarditis		
Mentions 2 further side effects including: weight gain, constipation, dry mouth, flu-like symptoms, nausea, sleepiness, dizziness		
Explains need for regular blood tests (once weekly for 18 weeks, every 2 weeks for a year then once monthly thereafter) to monitor WCC		
Explains must avoid drinking alcohol and caffeine		
Stresses importance of compliance and must not stop suddenly and to inform medical staff if they have missed a dose		
Safety netting - Informs to seek immediate advice if any adverse side effects or takes too many tablets		
Advises to seek medical help immediately if they develop a sore throat (due to risk of agranulocytosis)		
Explains they start at a low dose and slowly up-titrate dose		
Offers patient leaflet/information		
Summarises consultation		

Builds rapport with patient		
Avoids medical jargon		
Clear and concise		
Examiner's Global Mark	/5	
Actor / Helper's Global Mark	/5	
Total Station Mark	/30	

Learning Points

- Clozapine is an atypical antipsychotic only given if 2 other anti-psychotics have been trialled and have either been ineffective or if the patient develops a tolerance.

- Agranulocytosis is a potentially life-threatening side effect and will develop in 1-2% of patients, in a dose independent manner. Full blood count must be performed weekly for the first eighteen weeks, fortnightly for a year, and then monthly thereafter. The Clozapine Patient Monitoring Service (CPMS) keeps a close track of all patients on clozapine and will only allow for its release by pharmacy if the full blood count is normal.

- Despite the extensive side effect profile, clozapine is a very effective drug and one third of patients with chronic schizophrenia respond to treatment within 6 weeks and two thirds within a year.

1.16 "Healing hands"

Candidate's Instructions:

A 20-year-old lady called Summer has been admitted to the inpatient psychiatric unit following some unusual and reckless behaviour.

You are the foundation doctor based on the ward and have been asked by your consultant to take a history from the patient.

You have 7 minutes to take a history, after which you will be stopped and asked to present your findings and suggest an initial management plan.

Examiner's Instructions:

A 20-year-old lady called Summer has been admitted to the inpatient psychiatric unit following some unusual and reckless behaviour.

The foundation doctor based on the acute psychiatry ward has been asked to take a history from the patient.

At 7 minutes, please ask the candidate to summarise the case, and then ask the following three questions:

1. What do you think is the most likely diagnosis for this patient? (Bipolar affective disorder)
2. What differential diagnoses would you also consider?

3. What would you like to include in your initial management plan?

Actor's Instructions:

Background
You are a 20-year-old university student called Summer who was brought to the emergency department by your parents following a period of unusual behaviour. You were subsequently admitted to the acute psychiatric ward under Section 2 of the MHA (1983).

Your behaviour
You cannot keep still, and often lean close to the doctor in rather a provocative manner. At times you offer to place your healing hands on their body. At other times you get up and pace around the room in an excited manner. Your eye contact is very intense and your facial expression appears euphoric.

Your rate of speech is very fast and loud. At times it is difficult for the doctor to get a word in edge-ways and you often go off on a tangent about other topics which don't relate to the question you were originally asked. At times you may respond to messages from God that you are being sent. You get irritated when the doctor tries to bring you back to the subject. You are easily distracted.

Your history of symptoms
Over the past few weeks you have become more and more irritated by your family members who are always trying to "cramp your style". Lately you have been feeling happier than you have ever felt in your life with a great deal of energy, but for some reason your family seem worried and forced you to come to the emergency department. You think they are jealous of your "healing powers."

You are relishing student life and share a house with several other psychology students. Lately you have been feeling so excited that you haven't slept for several days. You are up all night writing long essays about your powers. Your mind races with fantastic ideas. You have an insatiable appetite. You are feeling more confident in your looks than ever before, and love wearing skimpy outfits as you love the attention you get. You have spent all of your student loan and savings on new clothes, jewellery and make up. You have slept with several different men over the last few days, some of whom you met when "out and about". You feel "in love" with the world and give out money to anyone you think may need it. You're not interested in drugs or alcohol as these would just "slow you down". You can see the TV in 3D and have x-ray vision which allows you to see inside people's bodies. This allows you to be a healer and you believe that this is a power that has been bestowed on you by 'God'. You are feeling incredibly optimistic and know that you have been 'blessed' with the ability to heal all suffering in the world. God is sending you messages, telling you to use your healing powers on everyone you meet.

On one occasion you were picked up by the police because you were using your healing powers on people at the local shopping centre. The Police didn't understand that you have special powers. You were released after questioning and do not have a criminal record.
Yesterday you splashed out on a brand new car using your credit card as you have spent all your savings. You drove several hours from university and dropped in on some family friends in the middle of the night to tell them about your special powers and to heal them of their health problems. It must have been them that called your parents.

You have no medical problems that you know of and don't take any regular medications. If asked, you admit that in the past you have had periods of feeling very low in mood to the point where you haven't wanted to leave the house for several weeks. Last year you were briefly admitted to hospital due to feeling suicidal and taking a paracetamol overdose. You think this was mainly due to a break-up with your boyfriend. You are therefore particularly enjoying the way you feel at the moment and have no insight that your current mood could in fact be pathological. You can't understand why your parents are so worried about you and you describe your mood as "fantastic". You have no thoughts of suicide of self-harm at present. You are adamant that you don't need any medication as "feeling this good can't be a bad thing".

If asked about your personality before the depression, you say that your mum has always called you "over emotional" since you were a child. However, you have had a happy childhood and have not experienced abuse of any sort. Your mum tells you that you had an aunt who "wasn't right in the head" and committed suicide when she was in her 40's.

BIPOLAR AFFECTIVE DISORDER STATION OSCE – "Healing hands"

Task:	Achieved	Not Achieved
Introduces self		
Clarifies to whom they are speaking and gains consent for interview		
Elicits history in a concise manner: Onset of behavioural change Possible triggers e.g. lack of sleep or life events Impact on daily life (e.g. work, studies, finances, relationships) Change in sleeping/eating patterns		
Explores risk-taking behaviours/vulnerability (such as sex with strangers, excessive spending, sexual disinhibition)		
Elicits psychotic symptoms (delusions of grandeur/special powers, thought interference, religious preoccupations)		
Excludes suicidal ideation/thoughts of self-harm (Performs basic suicide risk assessment)		
Enquires about the patient's social situation (e.g. source of income for current spending pattern, living arrangements etc.)		
Enquires about forensic history/involvement with the Police		
Asks about personal history (childhood, relationships, education) and pre-morbid personality		
Asks about past medical history		
Asks about past psychiatric history		
Asks about regular medication and allergies		

Excludes illicit substance use and alcohol use		
Asks about family history, including mental health issues		
Explores insight into present mental state and behaviour		
Summarises and presents findings concisely		
Correctly identifies the diagnosis (bipolar affective disorder)		
Offers at least two other differential diagnoses including: schizophrenia, schizoaffective disorder, personality disorder, ADHD, stimulant substance abuse or endocrine disturbance		
Explains basic steps for management Drug therapy (Antipsychotics in acute episodes and mood stabilisers for prophylaxis e.g. lithium) Psychotherapy		
Employs a professional and calm approach		
	/20	
Examiner's Global Mark	/5	
Actor / Helper's Global Mark	/5	
Total Station Mark	/30	

Learning Points

- According to the ICD-10 criteria, a diagnosis of Bipolar Affective Disorder (BPAD) can be made when there have been at least two episodes of significant mood (depressive, manic or hypomanic) and behavioural disturbance. At least one of these episodes must be manic or hypomanic.

- Manic episodes differ from the hypomanic type in that there are particularly severe (therefore having an impact on relationships, work, studies etc.) and involve psychotic symptoms.

- It is important to remember that BPAD carries one of the highest lifetime risk for suicide attempts and suicide completion of all psychiatric illnesses. Lithium has been shown to reduce this risk.

1.17 "Insomniac"

Candidate's Instructions:

You are a foundation doctor working in a GP practice. A 30-year-old woman called Liberty has presented to your clinic because she is having difficulty sleeping and would like some sleeping tablets.

Please perform a full Mental State Examination with a view of establishing a likely diagnosis. You do not need to take a detailed history.

You have 7 minutes to perform the examination; after which the examiner will ask you to present, and then discuss your findings.

Examiner's Instructions:

A young woman of 30-years called Liberty has presented to the GP practice today as she been experiencing difficulty sleeping. The foundation doctor at the practice has been asked to spend seven minutes performing a Mental State Examination.

Please stop the examination after seven minutes and ask them to summarise their findings.

After this please ask the candidate the following questions:

1. What do you think is the most likely diagnosis for this patient? (Generalised anxiety disorder)

2. What differential diagnoses would you also consider?

3. What would you like to include in your initial management plan?

Actor's Instructions:

Background – You are a 30-year-old woman who has presented to the GP practice with difficulty sleeping. Your expectation is to get some sleeping tablets.

This is a Mental State Examination, so the candidate should not be focusing on a detailed history. However, if they ask you have no medical conditions or previous mental health problems, and neither does your family. You do not take any regular medications, illicit drugs or alcohol, and rarely drink coffee.

Below is a break-down of your "mental state" for this station:

MSE component	Description
Appearance and Behaviour	you look well, appropriately and smartly dressed and well-groomed. You are rather fidgety and look down at your lap a lot. You are slightly tremulous and your facial expression is tense
Speech	Your speech is quiet, but of normal rate, quantity and tone
Mood	Your affect is slightly flattened, but you are not tearful. You describe your mood as "fine". If asked, you admit that you feel anxious most of the time and have been this way for as long as you can remember. Your appetite is decreased of late and if asked, you say that this is because of butterflies in your stomach and often have to "dash to the loo", especially when at work. Your sleep is poor. You lie awake for hours and notice that your heart races
Thought	Process– Your answers are coherent, relevant and appropriate. You don't veer off topic. If you are asked – no-one is interfering with your thoughts Content– You are not having any thoughts that are delusional in nature. If asked, deny any strong religious beliefs or convictions. You don't have any suicidal thoughts, intentions or any feelings of worthlessness. Although sometimes you wish you could be more like other people who 'don't get so worried about things.' If asked about feelings of anxiety, you explain that you constantly worry

	about a whole range of things including issues at work, your physical appearance, and personal relationships (i.e. without specific triggers). You are worried that your lack of sleep is affecting your performance at work. If asked, you don't have any particular phobias. You don't have any recurrent intrusive thoughts that are out of context with your beliefs, or any urges to perform rituals such as hand-washing or checking. You have not experienced fear of leaving the house or social situations
Perception	You are not seeing or hearing anything that other people cannot
Cognition	You have not felt confused or disorientated at any point. However, if asked, you have noticed that your concentration is poor, particularly at work.
Insight	if asked whether you think that your behaviour is unusual, you should admit that you are a "bit of a worrier" and have always been this way. You are aware that others around you don't get as "hung up" on issues as much as you do. You are keen to get help if offered, and hope that a sleeping pill will help "stop me worrying so much."
Risk	You have had fleeting thoughts of ending it all when it becomes too much, but have not made any plans, preparations, and do not feel you would go through with such a thing

Psych OSCE – "Insomniac"

Task:	Achieved	Not Achieved
Introduces self and clarifies whom they are speaking to		
Explains the nature of the interview and gains consent		
Comments on appearance		
Comments on behaviour		
Comments on speech		
Comments on objective mood		
Comments on affect		
Comments on subjective mood		
Enquires specifically about suicidal thoughts and risk		
Comments on thought form		
Comments on thought content and phobias		
Comments on visual hallucinations		
Comments on auditory hallucinations		
Comments on cognition		
Comments on level of insight "do you think you worry about things more than others? do you think this is having an impact on your life?"		
Elicits information sensitively and appropriately		
Summarises findings in a structured, logical manner		
Gives a primary diagnosis of GAD and two sensible differentials (panic disorder, social phobia, hyperthyroidism, stimulant abuse, alcoholism, etc.)		

Offers a suitable medical management plan; full medical examination, investigations including baseline observations, blood tests (such as U+Es, TFTS, Cortisol) to exclude organic causes, ECG if having palpitations/racing heart		
Offers a suitable psychiatric management plan: self-help, psycho-educational groups, CBT, pharmacological therapy such as SSRIs.		
	/20	
Examiner's Global Mark	/5	
Actor / Helper's Global Mark	/5	
Total Station Mark	/30	

Learning Points

- Diagnosis of generalised anxiety disorder requires the exclusion of other forms of anxiety such as panic disorders (e.g. agoraphobia) and phobias (e.g. social phobias) which have specific triggers. It is also important to rule out OCD by excluding repetitive obsessive thoughts or ritualistic behaviour.
- Generalised anxiety is associated with persistent feelings of anxiety/worry which are present for most, or even all of the time without a specific trigger.

- It is also crucial to exclude medical causes for anxiety related symptoms such as a racing heart and tremors (e.g. hyperthyroidism, hypoglycaemia, illicit substance/stimulant use and alcoholism).

- Risk factors include female gender, being aged between 35 and 54, divorced/separated and living alone/social isolation.

- Screening tests such as Beck's Anxiety Inventory can be a useful diagnostic aid.

1.18 "To balance out your hormones"

Candidate's Instructions:

A 30-year-old lady called Charmaine has been admitted to the inpatient psychiatry ward following her first episode of mania. The consultant wants to start her on lithium to help stabilise her mood.

You are the foundation doctor based on the acute psychiatry ward. Your colleagues have taken a thorough history and Mental State Examination (MSE) and you have been asked to counsel the patient about initiating lithium therapy.

She is an informal patient and has been judged by the consultant to have capacity to consent to medication. You have 7 minutes for your discussion.

Examiner's Instructions:

A 30-year-old lady called Charmaine has been admitted on the inpatient psychiatry ward following her first episode of mania. The consultant wants to start her on lithium to help stabilise her mood.

The foundation doctor based on the acute psychiatry ward has been asked to counsel the patient about starting this drug. She is an informal patient and has been judged by the consultant to have capacity to consent to medication.

Pay particular attention to the candidates use of medical jargon

Actor's Instructions:

Background
You are a 30-year old lady called Charmaine who has recently been admitted to the inpatient psychiatry ward following your first episode of mania. During this episode you went on a huge gambling spree and spent your entire life savings, you became socially and sexually disinhibited and aggressive towards family members and friends.

Your consultant has recommended initiating lithium therapy. The foundation doctor on the ward would like to talk to you about starting this new medication. Your current mental state is calm and lucid and you are able to take in and weigh up the information given.

You don't know anything about the drug and have never heard of it before, however are keen to find out as much as possible to help you make your decision and help you get back to your job as a teacher.

You are in a long-term relationship and are planning on having children in the near-future, although you're not currently "trying". This is something that is very important to you. If the candidate mentions any potential risks to a developing baby, you are shocked.

You have no physical health concerns other than mild asthma, and you have no known allergies. You are not on any regular medications, except for a salbutamol inhaler which you rarely use. You have a family history of hypothyroidism on your mother's side and your father had an MI aged 50. You have never smoked, drink 2 to 3 glasses of wine a week and have never taken any illicit drugs.

MEDICATION STATION OSCE – Lithium counselling

Task:	Achieved	Not Achieved
Introduces self, clarifies to whom they are speaking		
Explains the purpose of the discussion and gains consent to proceed		
Explains the benefits of lithium treatment (mood stabilisation)		
Explains that lithium is taken once a day, usually at night		
Discusses common side effects (such as weight gain, tremor, metallic taste, nausea, vomiting)		
Explains that most side effects can be treatable (e.g. propranolol for tremor, healthy diet and exercise for weight gain)		
Explains need for baseline tests (U&Es, TFTs, ECG)		
Explains need for long-term blood monitoring (TFTs, U&Es and lithium levels)		
Explains risks of teratogenicity (such as congenital cardiac abnormalities)		
Describes the signs of toxicity (worsening side effects as above plus ataxia, reduced consciousness, myoclonus, seizures)		
Explains risk of sudden cessation of the drug (may cause mania)		
Asks about current medication		
Checks for drug allergies		
Asks about alcohol use (when taken with lithium can cause drowsiness/cognitive impairment)		
Asks about past medical history		

Asks about family history (such as thyroid, renal or cardiac disease)		
Gives the patient an opportunity to ask questions		
Counsels the patient in a clear and concise manner		
Offers an information leaflet		
	/20	
Examiner's Global Mark	/5	
Actor / Helper's Global Mark	/5	
Total Station Mark	/30	

Learning Points

- Lithium can be extremely effective in stabilising mood in acute mania and in the prevention of recurrence. It has also been shown to reduce suicide risk both in bipolar and unipolar depression.

- Remember the '4 T's' of Lithium side effects: Tremor, Thirst, thyroid dysfunction and teratogenicity.

- If levels and side-effects are not closely monitored it can lead to renal and cardiac damage, and in severe cases can cause lasting cognitive and cerebellar dysfunction. Careful counselling including contraception advice is therefore essential.

1.19 "Colleague Concerns"

Candidate's Instructions:

You are the foundation doctor working on the Endocrine ward. Over the past few weeks, you have noticed that Paul, one of the senior nurses you work with has become more withdrawn and has been behaving strangely. Today, when asking him about a patient's discharge plans, he becomes tearful. You have taken him aside to talk about his feelings.

You have 7 minutes to take a psychiatric history from Paul, after which you will be asked to summarise the case and evaluate his risk.

Examiner's Instructions:

A 29-year-old nurse called Paul has been acting more withdrawn at work and the foundation doctor has been become concerned regarding his behaviour. They have been asked to take a psychiatric history and evaluate risk.

After 7 minutes stop the candidate and ask them to summarise their findings. Once complete ask the following questions:

1. How would you rate this patient's suicide risk?
2. What aspects of his case led you to give him this risk rating?

Actor's Instructions:

Background and behaviour:
You are a 29-year-old senior nurse called Paul working on the Endocrine ward. You have recently had an incident where a colleague posted an insulting image on your Facebook account saying that you were a 'home-wrecker'. This is the first time anyone has asked you about your feelings and you are willing to share it. You make little eye contact and speak in a detached manner.

History of symptoms:

You have had 3 very rocky relationships with members of staff over the past 2 years which has led to you being alienated from the other nurses and gossiped about. One of these relationships provoked a divorce between two senior doctors who have been working at the hospital for many years.

You feel isolated and that no one likes you. You have not been sleeping well and have been taking lorazepam and anti-histamines which you have stolen from the drugs cupboard. You have been drinking a bottle of wine a night to help 'ease the pain'. You do not take recreational drugs.

You were diagnosed with anxiety and depressive disorder as a teenager. You have been in admitted to the psychiatric unit for taking a diazepam overdose when you were 21 following breaking up with a boyfriend. You were glad at that time to have survived. You have no history of self-harm. You have difficulty making friends at work and live far away from your family and old university friends. You have no past medical history or regular medication.

Your self-esteem is rock bottom, and the only thing you enjoy is looking after your patients. You have found it very difficult to remember jobs however, and over the past week there have been errors in patient care. For example, you gave one patient another patient's medication as they shared the same surname. You became tearful because you have forgotten that patient A was going home and that you have not prepared transport. You have no history of hallucinations or delusions.

When asked about suicide you explain that all this pain you feel is not worth being 'in this reality' and that you would rather be 'on the other side.' You have gathered a supply of lorazepam at home which would be enough to end your life. You have not written a suicide note or made a will because 'who will care to read it?' You think you'll take the pills when you have driven to a secluded area in the nearby national park so that no one will find you. You have thought about doing this in the next few days.

SUICIDE RISK STATION OSCE - Worried Colleague

Task:	Achieved	Not Achieved
Introduces themselves and establishes rapport		
Elicits history of presenting complaint from patient in a concise manner		
Asks about depressive symptoms		
Asks specifically about current suicidal ideation		
Asks about self harm		
Elicits the patient's isolation		
Asks about plans for suicidal act and the future		
Asks about a suicide note/financial planning		
Asks about precautions against being found		
Elicits suicide plans are premeditated rather than impulsive		
Asks about alcohol and substance abuse		
Asks about past psychiatric history		
Asks about past medical history		
Asks about medication		
Asks about anxiety symptoms		
Rules out psychosis		
Summarises consultation fluently		

Advises that the patient is high risk of suicide		
Gives examples of what determines the patient at being high risk (male, single, isolated, previous attempts, history of depression and anxiety, alcohol use, health care worker, plans for future attempts)		
Non judgmental approach		
Examiner's Global Mark	/5	
Actor / Helper's Global Mark	/5	
Total Station Mark	/30	

Learning Points

- Knowing the suicide risk stratification is essential at determining level of risk and need for further management. A usual acronym is SADPERSONS (Juhnke, 1994 and Patterson et al. 1983)

- S - Male sex
  - Age <18 and >50
    D - Depression
    P - Prior history of attempts
    E - ethanol/drug use
    R - Rational thinking loss (psychosis/organic disorder)
    S - Social Support (lack of)
    O - Organised plan
    N - No spouse/significant other
    S - Sickness (medical/psychiatric co-morbidities).

- Mental illness can affect anyone including members of staff around you. As a medical professional it might only be you that has noticed a member of staff that is of high risk. As soon as this is identified, senior support is essential at managing these cases appropriately and safely.

- The ethical dilemma comes from breaking confidentiality in order to take the patient out of the working role to gain appropriate mental health support. Clearly in this case, some members of the nursing staff are not providing the patient with support and are provoking their low mood. Therefore, the patient should be asked who is a trusted member of the senior nursing team to be informed.

- Health care professionals are at a high risk category of suicide and mental illness. There is often fear arising from disclosing mental illness on the implications it has on employment. However, according to the GMC, if a doctor is open about their illness and seeks means to have it well controlled it will not affect future employment.

1.20 "The icecaps"

Candidate's Instructions:

You are a foundation doctor working in busy district general hospital emergency department. You have been asked to see Harrison, a 26-year-old male who presented today at the request of his girlfriend who is concerned over some recent 'erratic' behaviour.

He has a past medical history including depression and anxiety disorder.

Please take a brief history and perform a Mental State Examination (MSE). You have 5 minutes after which the examiner will ask you to summarise your findings and formulate a differential diagnosis.

Examiner's Instructions:

A 26-year-old man called Harrison has presented to the emergency department at the request of his girlfriend who is concerned over his recent behaviour.

The candidate has 5 minutes to take a focused history and conduct a Mental State Examination (MSE).

At 5 minutes please stop the candidate, ask them to summarise their findings, present the MSE, and give a differential diagnosis.

Actor's Instructions:

Background:
You are a 26-year-old man called Harrison who has come to the emergency department with your worried girlfriend. You are wearing a black t-shirt and dirty jogging bottoms. Your hair is unkempt. You maintain eye contact. You are intermittently quite restless and fidgety. Your speech is low in tone and you take long pauses before answering questions.

History of symptoms:
Over the past two months, you have noticed a change in the way you feel and see the world. You have become pre-occupied with thoughts about climate change and the inevitable apocalypse. This came about when a customer came into your butcher's shop and left a newspaper containing a worrying article about the state of the polar icecaps. It was at this point you realised you'd left your lights on in your bedroom. This was therefore the cause of the icecaps melting. You feel solely responsible for climate change, and know you are singly responsible for the impending apocalypse. You are naturally feeling guilty and worried about this, to the point where you have been having trouble sleeping. You have also found your appetite has been poor which is a good thing because "did you know that cattle are a big contributor to climate change?"

Your girlfriend has no idea how severe the state of the planet has gotten and you find this immensely frustrating. Sometimes you have very angry verbal outbursts at her. You have grown more distant since your realisation, and you think she secretly hates you because of what you have done.

You are no longer interested in going to work and making a living. Your colleagues have said that they think you need a break to get your head around things, but they talk about you behind your back. You know it sounds crazy but sometimes you can hear what they have been saying as you fall to sleep; things like "he's so selfish/he's such an idiot/he should have been more careful/he's a waste of a life". Sometimes, you have to listen music and drink alcohol in order to distract you from their voices. You drink 4 cans of strong lager every night.

Last year, you were diagnosed with mixed depression and anxiety disorder for which you almost required hospitalisation if you had not responded to the second medication they started you on. The episode lasted around 2 months and then you didn't need the medication anymore so stopped taking it. You have a past medical history of ulcerative colitis for which you take mesalazine twice a day. You have no known drug allergies. Your mother has generalised anxiety disorder.

You are aware that you are depressed and anxious but you can't help it when you've caused such a huge problem. All of humankind will know your name as the man who caused the apocalypse. If it wasn't for your girlfriend, you would have taken your life out of shame. You have no suicidal ideation or plans at present.

MSE station – 'The Icecaps'

Task:	Achieved	Not Achieved
Introduces self and checks identity		
Elicits history from patient in a concise manner		
Asks about depressive symptoms (e.g. low mood, low energy, insomnia/early morning wakening, poor appetite, feelings of worthlessness/hopelessness/helplessness)		
Asks about anxiety symptoms (e.g. pre-occupied with worries about the future, ruminating about past action, feeling guilty, sleep disturbance, feelings of panic, fear and uneasiness),		
Asks about past medical history		
Asks about medication history and allergies		
Asks about alcohol and drugs		
Asks specifically about current suicidal ideation/Brief suicide risk assessment		
Elicits that beliefs are fixed and delusional		
Asks about auditory and visual hallucinations		
Accurately describes **appearance and behaviour** as being unkempt, keeps good eye contact, restless		
Describes **speech** as being low in tone, volume and rate.		

Describes **mood and affect**: mood is anxious and depressed while affect is incongruous more depressed than anxious.		
Describes evidence of psychosis including auditory hallucinations for abnormal **perception.**		
Thought form: offers that the patient takes a long time to formulate thoughts with their long pauses between answering questions. (This implies psychic retardation) **Thought content**: fixed beliefs/pre-occupation/over-valued ideas (e.g. that they are solely responsible for the the apocalypse or that the apocalypse is actively occurring despite evidence against this).		
Cognition: patient is orientated to place, time and person.		
Insight: explains the patient has insight into the auditory hallucinations "being crazy" but has no insight around his delusion of being the sole cause of the apocalypse/apocalypse occurring.		
Accurately offers differential as psychotic depression and any one other of (schizophrenia, drug induced psychosis, bipolar disorder, obsessive compulsive disorder).		
Non judgmental approach		
Empathetic manner		
Examiner's Global Mark	/5	
Actor / Helper's Global Mark	/5	
Total Station Mark	/30	

Learning Points

- Delusions and hallucinations in psychotic depression tend to be congruous to the mood states. For example, the content of hallucinations is often scathing or belittling of that individual.

- Patients with psychotic depression tend to have more insight into the nature of their hallucinations being unreal as compared to those with schizophrenia or psychotic disorder.

- Treatment of psychotic depression often requires a combination of antidepressants and antipsychotics. Patients are at very high risk of suicide and will often require hospitalisation. If they are refractory to medication ECT is often effective. A helpful acronym to remember symptoms of depression is CAGED IN

    C: poor Concentration
    A: reduced Appetite
    G: feelings of Guilt/worthlessness
    E: low self-Esteem/self-confidence.
    D: Direct self harm/suicide

    I: Insomnia/sleep disturbance
    N: No sex drive

1.21 "Antisocial and irritable

Candidate's Instructions:

A 17-year-old boy called Taylor has been brought into your GP surgery by his mother who is concerned that he is behaving oddly as he has become antisocial and irritable. His mother has decided not to be present during the consultation as she feels her son will be more open without her there.

You are a foundation doctor based at the GP practice and you have been asked to take a history from the patient.

You have 7 minutes to take the history, followed by 1 minute to summarise your findings and initial management plan back to the patient.

Examiner's Instructions:

A 17-year-old boy called Taylor has been brought into the GP surgery by his mother who is concerned that he is behaving oddly as he has become antisocial and irritable. His mother has decided not to be present during the consultation as she feels her son will be more open without her there.

The foundation doctor based at the GP practice has been asked to take a history and formulate a management plan and explain this plan to the patient.

At 7 minutes, if the candidate has not already done so, prompt them to summarise their consultation and discuss their management plan with the patient.

Actor's Instructions:

Background
You are a 17-year-old boy called Taylor of stocky build wearing jogging bottoms and a T-shirt. You have been forced to come to the GP by your mum who keeps nagging you for spending too time in your room and not joining the family at meal times.

Your behaviour
You are annoyed that you have wasted valuable time coming to the GP surgery in order to convince your mum that you are not abnormal. You are keen to get this consultation over with so that you can prove to her she is wrong. Throughout the consultation you are embarrassed and can easily become defensive saying "why does it matter?'

Your history of symptoms
You care about your body and appearance; you want to maintain good health and that is your priority at the moment. Sometimes you slip up and eat a little too much (you become a bit embarrassed when talking about this). You admit to eating up to 5 chocolate bars, 6 muffins and 5 donuts on the last occasion. During these periods you feel totally out of control. In order to compensate you have been doing exercises in your room.

Your daily exercise regime lasts 3 hours and 25 minutes: it involves running on the spot, skipping, star jumps, weights and other fat burning exercises. When asked what you eat normally you explain that you try to have a banana for mid-morning snack and porridge for lunch. Sometimes you do get hungry and then you have one of your *slip ups* but you always take laxatives following these episodes to help get rid of all the toxins which make you feel disgusting and fat. You'll then add an extra hour onto your training session the next day. You have been doing this up to 2-3 times a week for the last 6 months. Your mum doesn't believe any of this and is worried that you are always alone. She doesn't trust anything you're saying and it's not fair!

Otherwise you try to work hard at school but get easily distracted with gossip from other students. There's a girl you really like at school but you haven't had the confidence to ask her out as you want to get thinner first. You were bullied at primary school for a number of years about your weight. You do like learning, however, and hope to become a doctor someday but are not sure if you are clever enough and feel that you might not get into medicine if you're too fat. You insist that you do not take illicit drugs, smoke or drink alcohol. You are a little stressed at the moment with all that's going on. You don't sleep very well and have been waking up early in the morning but you have not had any thoughts of suicide and have never self-harmed. You do not have any previous medical history and have no family history of mental illness. You are not on any regular prescribed or OTC medications and have no known drug allergies.

Bulimia Nervosa STATION OSCE – 'Antisocial and Irritable'

Task:	Achieved	Not Achieved
Introduces self		
Clarifies who they are speaking to and gains consent		
Elicits history of presenting complaint with a focus on psychiatric history		
Establishes the nature of the eating disorder including binge eating, vomiting and purging.		
Asks about physical symptoms (palpitations, SOB, sweating, dizziness) and biological symptoms (weight changes, appetite, libido)		
Asks about past medical history		
Asks about past psychiatric history		
Asks about personal history (childhood, relationships)		
Asks about family history with focus on mental health and suicide		
Asks about drug history and allergies		
Asks about comorbid drug / alcohol misuse		
Asks about forensic history		
Risk assessment: suicide and self-harm risk, considers hospitalization if malnourished.		
Explains a differential diagnosis to patient using lay terms: likely bulimia nervosa with aspects of anorexia nervosa and/or muscle dysmorphia		
Further investigations: BMI, FBC, iron studies, cortisol, TFT, U+E's including PO3+ and Mg2+, ECG		
Offers treatment such as family psychotherapy and CBT. SSRI's may be indicated if severe.		
Discusses how best to tell family		
Offers a second consultation as follow-up		
Clear and concise consultation		
Non judgmental approach		
Examiner's Global Mark	/5	
Actor / Helper's Global Mark	/5	
Total Station Mark	/30	

Learning Points

- Use the SCOFF criteria for an easy way to remember the questions you should ask when considering an eating disorder:

    SCOFF
    Sick: have you ever made yourself sick? (remember to ask about other compensatory behaviours such as over exercise and laxative abuse)
    Control: have you ever had a feeling of loss of control when you eat?
    One stone: have you lost/gained weight?
    Fat: Do you feel fat?
    Food: does it dominate your life?

- Muscle dysmorphia, (AKA bigorexia) is a recently acknowledged body dysmorphic anxiety disorder associated with a preoccupation of increasing muscle mass and a delusion that muscles are too small. Much like bulimia, this disorder is associated with a poor self-esteem. The disorder can interfere with ALD and patients may prioritize weight lifting and exercise over their family, social life and work commitments. This condition is seen as similar to anorexia in that there is body dysmorphia and obsession with body shape. This condition is associated with anxiety and depression and there is an increased suicide risk and risk of self-harm.

- Sometimes it is best to see adolescence without their parents to enable them to express themselves fully and to prevent conflict from interfering with the consultation. Always remember to do what is best for the patient.

1.22 "The worrier"

Candidate's Instructions:

You are a foundation doctor currently working in General Practice.

A 62-year-old retired GP receptionist called Tracey has come to see you at your GP surgery for some help. She has been getting anxious about leaving the house due to fear over urinary incontinence in public, and the embarrassment it would cause. She has never had any symptoms of urinary incontinence before, but has heard that it is something that happens as you get older. She has a friend who has tried Cognitive Behavioural Therapy for anxiety recently and is keen to find out if this is something that could help her.

You you have been asked by one of your colleagues to discuss CBT treatment with the patient.

You have 7 minutes for your discussion. Once the 7 minutes are over the examiner will stop you to ask some questions.

Examiner's Instructions:

A 62-year-old retired GP receptionist called Tracey has come to the GP surgery for some help. She has been getting anxious about leaving the house due to fear of becoming incontinent of urine in public, and embarrassing herself. She has never had any symptoms of urinary incontinence before but has heard that it is something that happens as you get older. She has a friend who has tried CBT for anxiety recently and is keen to find out if this is something that could help her.

The candidate is a foundation doctor based at the GP practice and has been asked to discuss CBT treatment with the patient.

At 7 minutes please stop the candidate and ask the following two questions:

1. Can you give me two examples of disorders where CBT has been shown to be effective?

    Answer: Depression, anxiety, eating disorders

2. What methods are you currently aware of for conducting CBT? How else can CBT be delivered?

    Answer: Individual sessions, Group sessions, online/e-learning, books

.

Actor's Instructions:

Background:
You are a nervous 62-year-old retired GP receptionist called Tracey. You are worried about leaving the house and going on long journeys as you have a fear that you might become incontinent of urine and that everyone will know.

Your behaviour:
You appear nervous and jittery. You apologize profusely for arriving a little late as it took you some time to work up the courage to leave the house. You ask where the nearest bathroom is just for 'peace of mind'.

History of symptoms:
You have never had urine incontinence before and have normal bladder control at present. You used to work in a different GP practice and used to come across patients with it all the time. You once saw a patient come into the practice with a wet patch down her leg and felt so terribly sorry for her, you didn't realize until then how easily these things can happen in normal every day women as they get older.

You have been to the GP a number of times to ask for something to prevent urine incontinence. You have been investigated for urinary incontinence and have now realized that it is not something you currently suffer from- but you are extremely fearful of this happening to you.

You have become so worried that you are avoiding leaving the house. Every time you even think about walking out you get palpitations, knots in your stomach and feel sick. You particularly avoid long journeys and never go anywhere without knowing if there is a toilet nearby. You do your food shopping online and have stopped going for coffee mornings with your friends. You go to the toilet 15-20 times per day to "check" you haven't wet yourself and you are now worried your family members are starting to take notice. Your neighbour invited you to a BBQ last weekend and you had to make an excuse not to go. Your daughter is getting married in Australia next year and you are worried you won't make the journey with all the long queues on the plane to get to the bathroom, and the long walks to toilets in the airport. That's not even including the wedding itself, what if you wet yourself in your dress? The mother of the bride can't be acting like that!

You have a friend who has tried CBT for anxiety and is keen to find out if this is something that could help you. They said that it is a talking therapy and you would like to know more about how it works. You become concerned if the doctor tells you that you would will be asked to face your fears and go out in public, and you worry that you will disappoint the therapist if you struggle to do so.

You have no past medical history except reflux, and are fully independent. You take omeprazole 40mg OD and are allergic to penicillin.

CBT counselling STATION OSCE – the 'worrier'

Task:	Achieved	Not Achieved
Introduces self		
Clarifies who they are speaking to and gains consent		
Elicits nature of anxiety		
Correctly elicits that the patients does not have any symptoms of incontinence		
Elicits patient's current knowledge about CBT		
Establishes how much/what specifically the patient wants to know about CBT		
Confirms that CBT is a talking therapy that is designed to look at how the patients thought patterns influence their behaviour, i.e.: "change the way you feel by changing the way you think"		
Explains that CBT is based on the theory that the disorder is not caused by past life events but the view the patient takes of them		
It uses problem solving methods to influence thought patterns		
Gives an example of this in relation to the patient's current problem		
The CBT therapist conducts an initial assessment with patient followed by 6-20 hour long sessions		
Discusses pros and cons to CBT such as helping develop proactive problem solving strategies but there is less focus on discussion around past life events and stressors. The patient may be given homework.		
Explores patient's concerns about CBT		
Explores patient's expectations from CBT		
Q1:CBT can be effective in anxiety, depression and eating disorders		
Q2: CBT is often delivered on a one to one basis but can be provided as a group session or in the form of books or online material		
Aids patient decision making by allowing her time to ask questions		
Facilitates an open discussion around the subject of CBT		

Avoids jargon and uses simple examples		
Gives information clearly and in a structured format		
Examiner's Global Mark	/5	
Actor / Helper's Global Mark	/5	
Total Station Mark	/30	

Learning Points

- Psychological therapies can be divided into:

    1. Social: such as family therapy or group therapy
    2. Supportive: reflection and emotional expression e.g. counselling
    3. Cognitive and behavioural: focus on changing negative thoughts and behaviours e.g. CBT
    4. Psychodynamic: unstructured- where the patient discusses what they wish to discuss to aid understanding of themselves. This allows patient to develop a relationship with therapist. This is used in complex personality disorders or long-term anxiety or depression.

- In specific phobias people learn to avoid their fears by operant conditioning- if they avoid their stimulus, their anxiety reduces. Avoidance behaviours are reinforced by a positive feeling of relief when specific fear is avoided. CBT acts to encourage patients to expose themselves to their phobias. Initially anxiety peaks but will eventually decrease with further exposure, in a process known as: "habituation."

- The theory behind CBT was developed by Aaron Beck in a series of papers in the 1960's. This outlined how some mental illnesses involved "cognitive distortions" (i.e. errors in the evaluation of information), and each of these distortions related to either the world, the self, or the future. These three areas were believed to be interconnected and formed the basis of "Beck's Triad" (Fig 1)

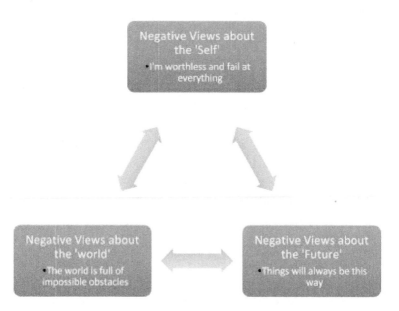

Fig 1. The features of Beck's Cognitive Triad

1.23 "Palpitations and sleep deprivation"

Candidate's Instructions:

A 32-year-old mother of 3 called Julia has attended GP surgery due to poor sleep and palpitations, and is seeking advice and treatment.

You are the foundation doctor based at the GP practice and have been asked to take a history. Please formulate a differential diagnosis and explain your management plan to the patient.

You have 7 minutes to take the history, followed by one minute to summarise your findings and initial management plan back to the patient.

Examiner's Instructions:

A 32-year-old mother of 3 called Julia has attended the GP surgery due to poor sleep and palpitations, and is seeking advice and treatment.

The foundation doctor based at the GP practice has been asked to take a history, formulate a differential diagnosis and explain their management plan to the patient.

At 7 minutes, if the candidate has not already done so, prompt them to discuss their differential diagnosis and management plan with the patient.

Actor's Instructions:

Background
You are a well kempt 32-year-old single mother of 3 children called Julia. You have come to the GP as you have been getting palpitations at night and are unable to sleep.

Your behaviour
You are initially quite timid and only give brief answers to questions. You then become tearful when questioned about your lack of sleep and begin talking about your home life.

Your history of symptoms
You have had these symptoms ever since your mother died 2 weeks ago. Your mother suffered from early-onset dementia and you were her main carer for the last 12 years of her life. She was a big part of your life and, even though her death was expected, it came as a huge shock you. Since her death you have felt alone and have become increasingly tearful. You keep thinking about her and find yourself hearing her voice sometimes. She has spoken to you a number of times since her death to offer comforting words and guidance. Hearing her voice is soothing but also makes you sad. You wonder whether this is normal or whether you are going crazy.

Your partner left you 6 months ago prior to your mother's death as he felt you were spending too much time looking after her. You were left with not only your mother to look after but 3 children under the age of 10. You work as an accountant for which you travel to the city 3 days a week and work from home the rest of the week. The children are in childcare when you do this. You have lost contact with the rest of your family and feel unable to cope with looking after the children, although this is always your priority above and beyond your own wellbeing. You enjoy your job but have found it increasingly difficult to concentrate at work recently and are worried that your boss has noticed.

You do not have any previous medical history and have never had suicidal thoughts or thoughts of self-harm. You are not on any regular or OTC medications and have no drug allergies. There is no family history of mental illness. You do not smoke, rarely drink alcohol and have never taken street drugs. Apart from sleep deprivation and palpitations you have not had any other physical symptoms.

Expectations from the consultation

You keep asking 'what is wrong with me Doctor?' and are keen for a medication that with help 'solve everything'. You are worried that hearing voices is abnormal and want to know if this makes you crazy. You are also concerned about childcare and being sacked from work due to other distractions.

BEREAVEMENT STATION OSCE – palpitations and sleep deprivation

Task:	Achieved	Not Achieved
Introduces self		
Confirms patient identity and gains consent		
Obtains a history of presenting complaint with focus on psychiatric history		
Establishes nature of hallucinations		
Asks about physical (chest pain, SOB, sweating, dizziness) and biological symptoms (weight changes, appetite, libido)		
Asks about past medical and psychiatric history		
Asks about personal history (childhood, relationships, occupation)		
Asks about family history with focus on mental health and suicide		
Asks about drug history, allergies and compliance, including comorbid drug / alcohol misuse		
Asks about forensic history		
Considers suicide and self harm risk		
Considers risk to the children – shows active concern about childcare		
Offers investigating organic causes e.g. TFTs, ECG		
Explains a differential diagnosis to patient: likely a normal bereavement process, possible underlying anxiety/depression		
Offers supportive management such as bereavement counselling and support services prior to considering medical treatment		
Suggests time off work/ working from home more often		
Suggests help with childcare		
Offers a second consultation as follow-up		
Addresses patients concerns		
Non judgmental approach		
Examiner's Global Mark	/5	
Actor / Helper's Global Mark	/5	
Total Station Mark	/30	

Learning Points

- There are 6 main stages of grief. These stages fluctuate in time-span and order and the bereaved may pass in and out of these stages as they progress through normal grief with mixed feelings and emotions.

  1. Shock/disbelief/numbness; anxiety, weeping, biological symptoms
  2. Anger; towards health care professionals caring for the deceased, friends/families for abandoning the diseased or towards the deceased themselves for no longer being around
  3. Searching/yearning; the desire to find the deceased. There may be vivid dreams or psuedohallucinations of the deceased with **preserved insight**
  4. Guilt; self blame for death, things that could have been done differently
  5. Sadness; biological and psychological features of depression
  6. Acceptance/letting go; hopes for the future, enjoyment of life and hobbies.

- Do a risk assessment: patients may be at risk of self-neglect, self-harm or suicidal ideation with the desire to join the deceased loved one.

- Adjustment disorder is characterized as an abnormal psychological response to a life stressor and can present as a mix of anxiety and depressive symptoms during bereavement. Antidepressants and further psychological therapies should be considered in this situation. However, patients progressing through normal grief usually require only non-pharmacological treatment such a bereavement counselling, childcare support or time off work. A short course of sleeping tablets could be considered if sleep deprivation remains ongoing.

1.24 "Not all it's cracked up to be"

Candidate's Instructions:

A 24-year-old new mother called Lily has come to see you at the GP surgery. She has a 1-week-old baby girl as is worried that she isn't being a "good enough" mother and wants some advice.

You are and foundation doctor based at the GP practice and you have been asked to take a history and formulate an initial management plan.

You have 7 minutes to take the history, followed by 1 minute to summarise your findings and initial management plan back to the patient.

Examiner's Instructions:

You are 24-year-old new mother called Lily of a 1-week-old baby girl has come to see the GP surgery as she is worried that she isn't being a "good enough" mother and wants some advice.

The foundation doctor based at the GP practice has been asked to take a history and formulate an initial management plan.

At 7 minutes, if the candidate has not already done so, prompt them to discuss their diagnosis and management plan with the patient.

Actor's Instructions:

Background
Your name is Lily and you are a slightly dishevelled 24-year-old new mother of a 1-week old baby girl. You have come to the GP as you feel totally inadequate as a mother and are unsure of what to do.

Your behaviour
You appear shy and avoid eye contact. You become tearful during the consultation when talking about the relationship you have with your baby.

Your history of symptoms
You are finding it difficult to enjoy the time you spend with your baby at the moment, as you feel isolated and alone. He cries constantly and you are exhausted. Being a mother is not all it's cracked up to be! You thought that having a baby would stop you feeling lonely and help you get your life back on track again. When your friends had babies they dressed them up in little outfits and they looked so cute and happy. You thought yours would be the same and that a baby would help you get closer to your family and friends but it's done just the opposite. You can't even breast feed properly as the baby won't latch on and feel totally incapable of caring for him. You are scared he might be losing weight. Your parents have only come to visit the baby once and are now off holidaying in the Caribbean. You've barely seen your friends this week as you've had to nap during the day most of the time when the baby finally rests. You've given up your dream job in media in order to care for your baby and are now regretting your decision to have a baby.

You deny auditory or visual hallucinations, and do not think anyone is interfering with your thoughts.

Your ex-partner, an avid businessman and the father of the child, left you a few months ago because he said you were hormonal and difficult to be with. He admitted, in a heated argument, that he didn't want to have a baby anyway and that it was a mistake. You thought that he might return once the baby is born but you haven't seen or heard from his since. Your friends all have supportive partners and families and it's completely unfair, all you wanted is to have a proper family just like everybody else and to be a good mother.

You feel lonely and simply tired of it all. You are worried that your resentment is having a negative impact on your relationship with the baby and feel guilty that you are becoming a bad mother. Despite this you always respond to your baby's cry's and feed, wash and change him as necessary. You have not had any thoughts of harming the child who is at home with a nanny, a family friend who is well known to you, that you hired temporarily. You have no thoughts of suicide and have never self-harmed. You have no thoughts to harm your baby. You do not have any previous medical history and have no family history of mental illness. You do not take illicit drugs, smoke or drink alcohol. You take no regular medications except for multivitamins.

Post Natal Low Mood STATION– not what it's cracked up to be

Task:	Achieved	Not Achieved
Introduces self		
Clarifies who they are speaking to and gains consent		
Elicits history of presenting complaint		
Establishes the nature of the postnatal low mood (onset, triggers, duration, timing)		
Asks about symptoms of depression (anhedonia, fatigue, lack of concentration)		
Asks about physical symptoms (palpitations, SOB, sweating, dizziness) and biological symptoms (weight changes, appetite, libido, sleep changes)		
Asks about psychotic symptoms (hallucinations, delusions, thought insertion, withdrawal, broadcast)		
Asks about past medical history		
Asks about past psychiatric history		
Asks about family history with focus on mental health and suicide		
Asks about drug history, allergies and compliance, including comorbid drug / alcohol misuse		
Asks about forensic history		
Risk assessment: suicide and self-harm risk		
Child safety assessment: asks about thoughts of harm to child, ensures baby is being looked after		
Explains a differential diagnosis to patient: likely postnatal low mood / baby blues.		
Further investigations: FBC, iron studies, cortisol, TFT, U+E's if she would like to investigate further		
Offers reassurance, does not offer pharmacological therapies		
Discusses ways to seek help with child support/ people to talk to such as midwife		
Offers a second consultation as follow-up to monitor for signs of postpartum depression		
Non judgmental approach		

Examiner's Global Mark	/5	
Actor / Helper's Global Mark	/5	
Total Station Mark	/30	

Learning Points

- The Baby Blues typically arises in the first 2 weeks postpartum and occurs in around 60% of mothers. There is little link with social variables. Mothers will be worried about inadequate mothering and be irritable and tearful as they adjust to the new role. It is important to reassure these women that the feelings should subside and offer a follow-up consultation if feelings continue beyond 2 weeks. It is best to avoid antidepressants in pregnancy and breastfeeding unless necessary as there may be adverse effects to the baby.

- Top tip; these patients can be extremely fragile and irritable, avoid confrontation and try to give them the support and confidence they need. They may be feeling guilty about their feelings towards their baby or inadequate as a mother. Acknowledge their feelings and try to reassure them that these are normal. Men can get this too so try to gauge the partner's thoughts and emotions towards the baby.

- The baby blues is usually self-limiting but around 1 in 10 mothers may go on to develop postpartum depression. This can be measured using the Edinburgh postpartum depression scale. Postpartum psychosis is rare but it is important to be aware of, these patients are usually hospitalized with their baby in specialist units.

1.25 DRABCDE "The rigid lady"

Candidate's Instructions:

You are a foundation doctor in the emergency department and you have been asked to examine a 48-year-old lady called Violet who came in via ambulance from the psychiatric inpatient unit.

You have been handed over by the paramedics that she has a diagnosis of schizoaffective disorder and she has recently been started on daily haloperidol injections.

She is unwell and is in Resus. You do not need to take a history. Please talk out loud during your examination.

You will be stopped after 6 minutes to give a diagnosis, initial investigations and a management plan.

Examiner's Instructions:

The candidate has been asked to examine a 48-year-old lady called Violet in the emergency department. The aim of the station is to test the candidate's ability to recognise neuroleptic malignant syndrome and its symptoms.

Please inform the candidate of their findings at their request, e.g. when looking at the patient from the end of the bed you can inform them that she is clammy and sweaty. Positive findings are listed below:

Danger: The patient is in the resus bed and you are safe to proceed

Response: The patient is drowsy. She is not responding to voice. But opens her eyes to her name

Airway: No snoring, swelling, stridor or evidence of airway obstruction

Breathing: Tachypneoic (respiratory rate 26), Sats 98% on 35% oxygen venturi, using accessory muscles to breathe, symmetrical chest expansion, chest clear.

Circulation: Pyrexic 39.5 degrees Celsius, Tachycardic (pulse 104), Hypotensive (blood pressure 94/50), Hot centrally and peripherally, capillary refill time <2 seconds, looks pale, sweaty and clammy. Incontinent of urine.

Disability: Confused GCS E3, V2, M5 10/15, lead pipe rigidity (increased tone) in upper and lower limbs, significant tremor in both arms

Everything Else: Abdomen soft and non tender, glucose 4.8.

Investigations include
- Bloods – FBC, U&E, calcium, LFTs, CK, INR – Sent for analysis
- ABG – pO2 24.4, pCO2 3.4 BE -4.5, Bicarb 16.0 Lactate 5.6
- Urinary drug screen – Sent for analysis
- CXR – Clear lung fields
- ECG – Sinus tachycardia Rate 110

Management includes
- IV Fluids
- Cooling – Take clothes off whilst maintaining dignity as much as possible
- Benzodiazapines if catatonic
- Doperminergic agents (however the evidence is limited and use is controversial)
- Stopping the offending medication is vital
- ICU referral If signs of respiratory distress, temp >40 or requiring sedation/IV cooling

Actor's Instructions:

You are a 48-year-old lady called Violet who is currently an inpatient in the mental health unit. You have schizoaffective disorder and have had multiple admissions to the mental health unit and tried many different antipsychotics. 1 week ago you were started on a new injection which was helping. Over the last 48 hours you have become very unwell. The candidate is a foundation doctor in the emergency department who has been asked to examine you.

You are sweaty, clammy and look unwell. You feel so ill that you can barely talk or move. You only make occasional groans and incomprehensible words in response to questions and you have your eyes closed unless spoken to. You are very confused about where you are.

Your arms and legs are so stiff they feel like lead pipes and you are hardly able to bend them. It takes quite a lot of force from the doctor to bend or move your arms and legs. Also you have a severe tremor in both of your hands. You are able to follow instructions but it takes a lot of effort for you to move.

You are heart is beating very quickly and your blood pressure has dropped. Your breathing is heavy and laboured. You have had some urinary incontinence but you are too confused to be embarrassed about it. Currently you are in a hospital bed in Resus and everyone is busy rushing around you and, understandably, you feel very distressed and are trying to take the oxygen mask off repeatedly.

EXAMINATION OSCE STATION- The rigid lady

Task:	Achieved	Not Achieved
Inspects surroundings/checks for danger		
Checks for patient response (patient is rousable)		
Introduces self		
Confirms patient name and DOB		
Gains consent		
Examines patient from end of bed		
Assesses airway		
Assesses breathing, offers to listen to the chest, asks for respiratory rate/oxygen sats		
Circulation – palpates pulse, asks for blood pressure/HR/Capillary refill time/listens to heart		
Asks for temperature		
Assesses mental state – AVPU or GCS		
Assesses tone and power of upper or lower limbs (examiner notes rigidity and tremor in both hands)		
Asks about/inspects for incontinence		
Palpates abdomen AND asks for glucose		
Summarises findings		
Gives correct diagnosis – neuroleptic malignant syndrome		
Gives appropriate differential diagnosis e.g. catatonia, malignant hyperthermia, serotonin syndrome or encephalitis/meningitis		
Lists appropriate initial investigations including any 4 of FBC, Blood cultures, CK, ABG, LFTs, U+E, clotting, ECG, CXR, consider LP/CT head		
Give appropriate initial management plan at least 2 of: Cooling, IV fluids, antipyretics, Senior review/ICU referral, consider benzodiazepines		
Explicitly asks for haloperidol to be stopped		
Examiner's Global Mark	/5	
Actor / Helper's Global Mark	/5	
Total Station Mark	/30	

Learning Points

- Neuroleptic malignant syndrome is a rare but life threatening reaction to neuroleptic medication, and is thought to be secondary to blockade of dopaminergic neurons. IT is typically caused by either antidepressants, anti-psychotics or anti-Parkinsonian medications.

- The four cardinal features are muscular rigidity (lead pipe), pyrexia >38C, autonomic instability and altered mental state. If the muscular rigidity is severe and sustained it can result in muscle breakdown (rhabdomyolysis) which is why creatinine kinase (CK) is an important investigation in their initial workup.

- Management is mainly supportive, ideally, in an ITU setting to prevent respiratory failure. The most important step is to stop all neuroleptic agents and typically patients will recover in 1-2 weeks unless they have been given a long acting depot, where it can last up to 3 weeks.

Old Age Psychiatry

2.1 "That thingamybob"

Candidate's Instructions

You are a foundation year doctor based at a GP surgery. A 78-year-old man called Albert has attended the practice. His daughter has recommended that he attends as he is becoming more forgetful.

Please take a history. You have 6 minutes to do so, after which you will be asked to summarise the findings and make an initial plan.

Examiner's Instructions

A 78-year-old man called Albert attends his GP surgery. He lives with his daughter and she encouraged him to make an appointment with his GP as she feels he has been more forgetful lately.

The foundation year doctor has been asked to take a history from the patient. Please stop the candidate after 6 minutes and ask them to make a summary, including a brief risk assessment, differential diagnosis, and an initial plan.

Actor's Instructions

Background:
You are a 78-year-old man called Albert and you have booked an appointment at the GP surgery because you have become more forgetful. You live with your wife and 45-year-old daughter who have both insisted you visit your GP.

History of symptoms:
Your memory problems initially started about 1 year ago when you noticed that it was difficult to find words. This has persisted, and over the past six months, your memory problems have got markedly worse. Your daughter had to remind you to visit the GP surgery today, as you completely forgot about it. You missed an appointment with the opticians and forgot to go to a friend's birthday party, which you feel embarrassed about. You've also noticed that you keep losing your keys and can never remember where you've put them. On one occasion you even left the taps running and the sink overflowed. Your daughter was very unhappy. On another occasion, an incident happened when your wife gave you your usual morning insulin injection, left for the shops, and your daughter nearly gave you the same dose again shortly after as you completely forgot you had already taken it. Luckily your wife returned before it was given and you didn't receive any extra insulin. Since then, your wife and daughter always check with eachother before giving your dose. This incident made you feel stupid, embarrassed and upset. But you know your family were just trying to look after you.

You used to be able to visit some friends nearby, but since you had a near-miss when driving, your wife doesn't want you to drive. You don't drive much, but sometimes you still use the car to go to the shops when your daughter or wife aren't around. You're starting to feel fed up and low, and think you're becoming a burden on the family. You used to enjoy playing bridge but now struggle to keep focused on the game. You've generally lost interest in your old hobbies and are struggling with disturbed sleep (waking in the night, restlessness). You now sleep in a separate room to your wife as she finds it so unsettling.

You have type 2 diabetes, high blood pressure and had a "mini-stroke" four years ago. You take some tablets for your blood pressure and diabetes, and insulin injections with your meals. You're drink an occasional shandy approximately every other evening and have never used recreational drugs. You used to smoke, but stopped 30 years ago. You smoked about 10 per day for 20 years. You have no history of mental health problems. You were reluctant to attend today but know that it is best to have things checked out.

Your mental state:
You are still eating well and you have not had any thoughts of suicide and wouldn't end your life, because of your family. You're very close to your wife and daughter and despite the issues with your memory there have not been any big arguments recently. You've never been aggressive or violent towards them. You have not had any paranoid thoughts of experienced any hallucinations. At the back of your mind you're worried because your dad had Alzheimer's disease.

Mark scheme - "That thingamybob"

Task:	Achieved	Not Achieved
Introduces self to patient		
Clarifies who they are speaking to and obtains consent		
Establishes rapport		
Establishes history of symptoms (nature, onset, timing, slow or step-wise, examples, exacerbating factors)		
Rules out physical causes (head injury, hypothyroidism, B12 deficiency, Parkinsonism, space occupying lesion)		
Asks about behavioural change (agitation, aggression, disinhibition, calling out)		
Asks about cognitive change (aphasia, apraxia, agnosia, planning and organising)		
Asks about depressive symptoms – (low mood, anhedonia, fatigue, sleep, energy levels, appetite, self-care)		
Asks about psychotic symptoms (delusions, hallucinations)		
Performs risk assessment, including dementia-related risk (wandering, leaving taps running / oven on, driving, neglect and asking specifically about suicidal ideation).		
Asks about past psychiatric history		
Asks about medical history, medication and allergies, compliance		
Asks about alcohol and drugs		
Asks about psychotic symptoms (hallucinations, delusions – particularly delusions of worthlessness, neglect etc.)		
Asks about family history		
Asks about social history (home support, type of accommodation, personal [self-care, dressing] and domestic [finances, cooking, cleaning] activities of daily living)		

Is sensitive towards patients concerns throughout, counsels patient appropriately		
Summarises consultation fluently, including risk		
Provides at least 3 possible differential diagnoses (E.g. Alzheimer's dementia, vascular dementia, Lewy Body Dementia, depression, hypothyroidism, B12 deficiency)		
Lists a plan: MMSE or Addenbrookes Cognitive Assessment (ACE), dementia bloods screen (FBC, U&Es, LFTs, TFTs, B12 and Folate), CT head, collateral history, memory clinic, functional assessment		
Examiner's Global Mark	/5	
Actor / Helper's Global Mark	/5	
Total Station Mark	/30	

Learning Points

- If you have ruled out delirium and suspect dementia, then perform a dementia screen. The purpose of this is to rule out reversible causes. This should include: FBC, U&Es, Calcium, Glucose, LFTs, TFTs, Serum Vitamin B12 & Folate.

- It is important to have an understanding of the stages of dementia, and the typical features of memory impairment as the disease progresses. Mild dementia is characterised by symptoms such as word-finding difficulties and misplacing objects. In moderate dementia patients can often become disorientated and go wandering from their homes and may become agitated or aggressive. Severe dementia is characterised by problems such as swallowing difficulties, incontinence and speech loss [1]. With these symptoms in mind, it is important to evaluate the level of risk by asking about common incidents such as wandering, leaving the oven on or taps running, and any acts of aggression.

- A common comorbidity of dementia is depression, and low mood or anhedonia can be a presenting symptom, often before memory problems are noticed. It is important to screen for symptoms of depression, as patients are likely to benefit from some form of anti-depressant treatment.

2.2 "The Good Wife"

Candidate's Instructions:

You are a foundation year doctor working on the acute medical unit (AMU). A 92-year-old man called Reggie has been admitted following a fall at home. His wife has felt that over the past few days he has becoming increasingly confused.

You have 5 minutes to take a collateral history from Mr Hammond's wife after which the examiner will ask you a series of questions.

Examiner's Instructions:

Reggie is a 92-year-old gentleman, his wife has come to visit him at the hospital and the candidate has been asked to take a collateral history.

At 5 minutes please stop the candidate and ask the following questions:

1. How would you classify Mr Hammond's confusion?

2. What might be causing his acute confusion/delirium?

3. What are some causes of chronic confusion?

4. How would you like to manage Mr Hammond's acute confusion?

Actor's Instructions:

Background:
You are a 70-year-old wife of Reginald "Reggie" (92 years old). Your name is Alexandra. You have come in today at the request of the medical team to give a summary of the events leading up to your husband's admission. You are wearing designer clothing, sunglasses and do not maintain good eye contact. You are impatient, appear bored and have a distaste for hospitals and the NHS in general.

History of symptoms:
The maid found Mr Hammond on the floor of the garage yesterday evening with a golf club in his hand. He was rousable but very confused. She called the ambulance who took him to the emergency department, where he was admitted under the medical team. Reggie has been behaving strangely for the past 2 to 3 days. He has been saying that the journalists have been writing about him, accusing him of unspeakable things. When asked what exactly, he gave a terrified, haunted look and hobbled off. He has been clutching his abdomen at times, and the maid said he was incontinent of urine, which is new. He had a hip operation 6 months ago and was recovering well with the help of Leon his private physiotherapist.

He has an irregular heart beat, benign prostatic enlargement and regularly suffers from constipation. He has no history of confusion and his memory is normally good. He has been taking co-codamol since the hip replacement, as well as rivaroxaban and tamsulosin daily and laxido as required.

He walks with one stick but is able to wander around the garden, with an exercise tolerance of 30 to 40 metres. He often spends his weekends at the local cricket club where he is the Senior President. On weekdays he reads in the library or at the members only whisky bar in town for which he is an honorary member. In other words, he does not show much excitement for time spent with you, and your relationship has become increasingly distant over the last 2 to 3 years.

The night before his admission you heard him rumbling around his bedroom, moaning and making an absolute racket throughout the early hours of the morning. In the afternoon the day after, Leon who had been visiting you socially, advised you to see if he was alright and he was fast asleep. On waking him he seemed to be quite lucid initially but then went back to that incessant rubbish about the newspaper journalists. He also called you Judie, the name of his vile, interfering daughter. The maid also noted that he needed help getting up from the toilet yesterday as his legs felt like jelly, and that she also noted incredibly strong smelling urine. He has eaten little in the way of food over the past few days and didn't drink his usual glass of whisky yesterday afternoon, which is unusual for him.

Does this mean that you should take control his health care as he now no longer has his mental faculties? You are very keen to let nature take its course. You don't think it would be fair to him - to prolong his life.

Delirium station - The Good Wife

Task:	Achieved	Not Achieved
Introduces the conversation		
Confirms relatives identify and gains consent		
Elicits history of symptoms in a concise manner (acute or chronic, timing, nature, onset, triggers e.g. change in medication)		
Elicits symptoms of delirium: agitation, disorientation to person		
Slowly progressive or step-wise		
Asks about delusions and hallucinations		
Asks about mood (low mood, anhedonia, fatigue)		
Asks about circadian rhythm disturbance		
Asks about recent falls or head injury		
Asks about recent infective symptoms: fever, cough, shortness of breath, urinary symptoms, frequency, urgency		
Asks about past medical history		
Asks about medication history and allergies		
Asks about baseline cognition		
Finds out about pre-morbid function (dressing, cooking, cleaning, mobility, finances)		
Asks about social history (alcohol, drugs, previous employment)		
Q: Defines confusion as a delirum/acute confusion		

Q: Acute causes (any three): Infective: UTI, LRTI, sepsis, encephalitis Metabolic/endocrine: electrolyte disturbance, constipation, urinary retention, AKI/uraemia, hypothermia, hypoxia, hypoglycaemia. Drug induced: Opiates (co-codamol), steroids Intracranial: Head injury, Chronic or acute subdural bleed, SAH, raised ICP.		
Q: Chronic causes: Dementias (Vascular/Alzheimer's/Lewy Body/Fronto- temporal Metabolic: Vitamin deficiency (Wernicke's Encephalopathy), hypothyroidism Psychiatric: Depression		
Q: Management. Conservative, medical and social domains (e.g. well lit area, investigating and treating the underlying cause, CT head, MDT approach including physiotherapy, social services and occupational therapy involvement)		
Non judgmental approach		
Examiner's Global Mark	/5	
Actor / Helper's Global Mark	/5	
Total Station Mark	/30	

Learning Points

- Delirium is defined as an acute, fluctuating change in mental status, disorganised thinking and altered levels of consciousness. It carries with it a high morbidity and mortality.

There are three main subtypes:
- Hyperactive: associated with high levels of arousal, agitation, hallucinations and delusions
- Hypoactive: associated with reduced energy, motor retardation and incoherent speech. Often overlooked as patients are quiet and do not draw attention to their behaviour.
- Mixed delirium

(Bestpractice BMJ: Delirium (2015))

- This case touches upon capacity and best interests. According to Good Medical Practice (GMC), in cases where patients do not have capacity around treatment choices, the clinician must consider the patient care their first concern. They must support and encourage the patient to be as involved as possible around treatment choices. They should consider if the capacity status is temporary or permanent. What treatment would provide overall benefit to the patient. Where there is a legally binding advanced statement/decision, the view of family members and close friends' should be considered.

- If there is disagreement between family/friends and the healthcare team, it can normally be resolved by a case conference/family meeting and involving senior members of the team. If despite these measures, the conflict remains, legal advice should be sought in making sure the best interests of the patient are met.

2.3 "A quick fix"

Candidate's Instructions:

You are a foundation doctor working in general practice. You have been asked to see Gary, a 69-year-old retired professional rugby coach. He has come in today to discuss various treatments for a recent diagnosis of depression.

Please explore his risk factors and discuss management strategies in a context of the biopsychosocial model for depression.

You have 7 minutes for your discussion. Once the 7 minutes are over the examiner will ask you some questions regarding the case.

Examiner's Instructions:

The candidate is a foundation doctor currently working in general practice. They have been asked to discuss the various treatment options and explore risk factors for depression with Gary, a 69-year-old retired rugby coach.

Please allow 7 minutes for the discussion. Once the 7 minutes are over please ask the following question:

"If Gary did not respond to initial treatment and stopped eating entirely due to his depression, what sort of treatment options would you then consider?"

Actor's Instructions:

Background:
You are a 69-year-old retired rugby coach called Gary. You have come in today to discuss the treatment options for your depression. The diagnosis was made by an the emergency department doctor you saw a week ago, when you attended with a 1-year history of poor sleep, lack of appetite and lethargy. You have come to terms with the diagnosis over the past week and are keen to hear the options of treatment. In general, you want a quick fix but also feel you can overcome the problems with 'mental resilience and distraction.'

History of symptoms:
Your biological risk factors for depression include a chronic illness: 'paroxysmal atrial fibrillation', for which you take a beta-blocker every morning. This has unfortunately stopped you from keeping up with your morning exercise regime that you have done since you were a professional rugby player. You decided to miss your cardiology clinic last week as you were too tired and didn't see the point as "nothing ever seems to get better."

When the doctor discusses antidepressant medication, you are very keen just to take the tablet and sort out the mood. You would like a quick fix. You have reservations however, about the risks of these medications in later life. Your older friend fractured his hip and the fall was due to 'too much medication'. You are keen to know what sort of side effects there are from these medications. Will this have any issue with your heart tablets? You are also inquisitive to how long they take to work.

The psychological risk factors you have include your tendency to brush your feelings under the carpet. Displaying emotion has always been a sign of weakness both when growing up, and at work as a rugby coach. You reflect on a moment of pride when you played the whole of a second half of a game with a fractured collar bone and did not notice until you finished. You see ignoring ailments as a sign of being tough. Your friends always disliked that you never wanted to discuss problems with them. They felt you let out the stress on your players when coaching.

When the doctor discusses cognitive behavioural therapy, you imagine this to be sitting on a sofa, analysing your dreams. After some explanation of the process you warm to the idea as improving coping strategies sounds like something you'd ask your players to do. But is it evidence based?

Your social risk factors include retiring 6 months ago, and moving to Somerset where your wife died suddenly of a heart attack 2 months later, at the age of 72. You have not managed to sell the house and move back closer to friends which is tough as you feel isolated and alone. You never had children.

Some strategies you have considered to improving your social life in Somerset is to volunteer as a rugby coach to the school in your local village. You have thought about this for sometime but never felt the energy to do so. You have no suicidal ideation or plans and have no psychotic thoughts or behaviours.

COUNSELLING A PATIENT ON TREATMENTS FOR DEPRESSION

Task:	Achieved	Not Achieved
Introduces the conversation		
Confirms patient identify and gains consent		
Establishes recent history of depressive symptoms from patient in a concise manner		
Asks about biological risk factors (e.g. chronic illnesses, family history, age)		
Recommends seeking treatment for atrial fibrillation (AF)		
Asks about psychological risk factors (coping with stress, life events – retired, wife passed away).		
Explores social risk factors for depression (e.g. social isolation, retirement)		
Establishes no suicidal ideation/psychotic symptoms		
Describes SSRIs as a treatment for depression and briefly describes its mechanism of action		
Explains that the effects of SSRIs do not occur straight away and it may take 2 weeks to see improvement in symptoms.		
Describes the side effects of SSRIs (any three of: dry mouth, headache, falls, hyponatraemia, drowsiness, GI disturbance, nausea, anxiety, erectile dysfunction, urinary retention, insomnia)		
Correctly reassures patient about no interaction between SSRI and beta blockers		

Concisely describes the approach of cognitive behavioural therapy (looking at the interaction between thoughts, feelings, behaviours and physical symptoms)		
Comments that CBT is an interactive exercise and requires its users to be keen to participate in a series of sessions either as a group, one to one or using computerised CBT		
Offers some other alternative therapy choices (e.g. mindfulness therapy, group therapy, psychotherapy)		
Offers some advice as to how to improve the patient's social network (e.g. join the rugby volunteer club)		
Advised that the patient should be referred to the Psychiatry team for assessment		
Consideration of other medications such as SNRIs or lithium (TCAs are contraindicated due to his AF).		
Explains that ECT is an option in such cases		
Non judgmental approach		
Examiner's Global Mark	/5	
Actor / Helper's Global Mark	/5	
Total Station Mark	/30	

Learning Points

- In the over 65 age group, careful consideration should be taken prior to starting an antidepressant medication. This is because of the prevalence of other co-morbidities such as ischaemic heart disease (IHD), cerebrovascular disease and polypharmacy. This increases the risk of drug-drug interaction and drug-disease interaction.

- All antidepressants are indicated in increasing risk of falls. In the elderly population, psychological therapies are recommended as first line or combination, unless severely depressed.

- Venlafaxine is a recommended treatment option in the management of treatment resistant depression. Elderly patients may take longer to respond to antidepressant treatment, making them easily labelled as having refractory depression.

2.4 "Run rabbit, run rabbit, run run run…"

Candidate's Instructions:

A 78-year-old man called Clifford has presented to the GP accompanied by his 45-year-old daughter. She is concerned that he has been 'out of sorts' recently.

You are the foundation doctor working at the GP surgery and have been asked to take a history from the patient.

You have five minutes to take your history followed by two minutes to perform an Abbreviated Mental Test Score (AMTS).

After 7 minutes you will have one minute to present your findings and formulate an initial management plan.

Examiner's Instructions:

A 78-year-old man called Clifford has come into the GP practice with his daughter. She is concerned that he has been 'out of sorts' recently.

The foundation doctor at the GP surgery has been asked to take a history from the patient and present their findings.

At 5 minutes stop the candidate and ask them to perform an abbreviated mental test score (AMTS).

At 7 minutes stop the candidate and ask them to: 'please present your history and formulate an initial management plan.'

At the end ask the candidate these questions:

1. What is the Most likely diagnosis?

2. What initial investigations would you perform?

3. What is your initial management plan?

Actor's Instructions:

Background
You are a 78-year-old man called Clifford. Your daughter has insisted that you come to see the GP today. You were at home this morning when she visited and she was concerned that you forgot to turn the hob off after you made breakfast. You have forgotten to turn the hob off 4 times in the past two months; you don't cook anymore and can't remember turning the hob on this morning. You think she is overreacting, as you would have realized the hob was on eventually and she should mind her own business.

History of symptoms
You have had some problems with your memory over the last 6-12 months, but you don't think it is anything out of the ordinary for your age. You often lose your keys, but think this is normal for anyone. If asked you have been locked out of your house several times recently, but your daughter keeps a spare set of keys. You sometimes forget your neighbour's names but you remember family members and do not forget faces.

Your daughter comes over to help you with cooking and cleaning as you have been getting slower at housework, she mentioned that sometimes when she comes over you seem confused for a few hours but then go back to normal. During these periods she said that you cannot remember her name or where you are. Your daughter keeps sending you to the GP, who often thinks you have a UTI, but the tests are always negative. You get defensive when asked if you can wash and dress yourself, and reject the idea that you need any help.

You have type 2 diabetes and high blood pressure for which you take Amlodipine OD and Metformin BD. Five months ago you got a dosset box to help you take your medication. You have been taken to the emergency department on 3 occasions after a fall at home, but you have never been admitted into hospital with any injuries. Over the last 2 months you have noticed you spill your tea more because you have shakes, your grandkids have said you are moving around slower as well. You do not drink or smoke, you've stopped driving 2 years ago after getting lost on your way home to the supermarket.

Your Mental State

Your appearance is unkempt and you have poor eye contact with the doctor. You are reluctant to talk to the doctor as you are upset to be there for no reason. You are rude to the doctor and threaten to leave the appointment. Your mood has been low for a long time, no suicidal thoughts. Your speech is slow and disjointed as you have difficulty remembering certain words. You see rabbits in your bedroom, your daughter claims to not see them, but you know they are there as they make noises eating their carrots under your bed. This keeps you up all night. You do not have insight to your condition – you think your daughter is overreacting and you want to go home.

AMTS

Name – Correct	Age – Incorrect
Date of birth – Incorrect	Time – Correct
Current monarch – Correct	Dates of WW1 – Incorrect
2 objects – Correct	2 people – Incorrect
Count backwards – Incorrect	Address – Incorrect

Total = 4/10

LEWY BODY DEMENTIA STATION OSCE - confused elderly patient

Task:	Achieved	Not Achieved
Introduces self		
Confirms patient identity and gains consent		
Elicits history from patient in a concise manner		
Asks about presenting complaint with an open question		
Asks about memory – short term memory, long term memory, names, faces		
Asks about onset and progression of symptoms e.g is it stepwise, gradual or sudden		
Asks about risky behaviour – wandering out, leaving the hob on, locking up		
Asks about triggers – illness, stroke, trauma, medications, seizures, bereavement, social stressors		
Asks about symptoms of low mood		
Asks about daily activities – washing, dressing, cooking, shopping, driving		
Asks about Parkinsonism symptoms – tremor, slow movements, difficulty writing/initiating movement		
Asks about hallucinations – Auditory or visual		
Asks about past medical history – diabetes, blood pressure, strokes, epilepsy, clotting disorders		
Asks about medication history and allergies		
Asks drug and alcohol history		
Conducts the AMTS exam fluently and correct score (4/10)		
Non judgmental approach		
QUESTION 1: Offers primary diagnosis of Lewy Body dementia and at least one other differential including		

Fronto-temporal Dementia, Alzheimer's disease, vascular dementia		
QUESTION 2: Investigations to rule out organic cause, confusion or dementia screen – urine dip, U+Es, TFTs, vitamin deficiencies, LFTs, CRP, Consider CT Head, MMSE		
QUESTION 3: Bio-psychosocial management. Conservative therapies – memory clinics, occupational therapist at home, education for family, Social services if care needs are not met, Referral to Parkinson's clinic if motor features are found. Medical management – Rivastigmine may help. Social support		
Examiner's Global Mark	/5	
Actor / Helper's Global Mark	/5	
Total Station Mark	/30	

Learning Points

- Assess the 5 A's of Dementia – agnosia, aphasia, apraxia, amnesia and abnormal behaviour.
- Be aware of how to differentiate between different types of dementia. The most common is Alzheimer's, but ensure you ask questions to rule out Vascular dementia (hypertension, diabetes, strokes, TIA, clotting disorders), Lewy Body Dementia (visual hallucinations, fluctuating symptoms, disrupted sleep-wake cycle, associated with Parkinsonian features) and rarer forms of dementia such as Fronto-temporal Dementia (disinhibition, personality and behaviour changes)
- Depression in the elderly can sometimes mimic dementia, cognitive decline can be seen with low mood. When the mood disorder is treated, cognition returns to normal
- Core features essential for diagnosis of probable LBD (Two needed for Diagnosis)

  Fluctuating cognition with significant variation in alertness and attention
  Recurrent florid complex hallucinations, often well formed and detailed (Visual 60%, auditory 20%)
  Motor symptoms of Parkinsonism (Bradykinesia, tremor and rigidity)

2.5 "Cameras and microchips.."

Candidate Instructions

You are a foundation year doctor working on an old-age psychiatric inpatient ward. Your consultant has asked you to review an 80-year-old patient called Tahir who was admitted last night.

Please perform a full Mental State Examination (MSE). Please do not take a history. You have 5 minutes to do this, after which you will be asked to present the MSE, perform a risk assessment, and provide a diagnosis.

Examiner's Instructions

An 80-year-old patient called Tahir was admitted to the old-age psychiatric inpatient ward last night. The ward consultant has asked the foundation year doctor to review them, summarise their Mental State Examination (MSE), and provide a differential diagnosis.

Please stop the candidate after 5 minutes, after which please ask the candidate the following questions:

1. Please present the MSE...
2. Please explain your risk assessment...
3. What do you think the most likely diagnosis is? (Dementia with psychosis)

Actor's instructions

Background

You are an 80-year-old Asian male called Tahir and have been detained under Section 2 of the Mental Health Act (1983). Police were called to your house because you were found wandering down a street erratically at 3:00am in your pyjamas. The Police stated that you were shouting at strangers, but you think this is an exaggeration.

This is a Mental State Examination, so the candidate should not take a history. You have past medical or psychiatric history. You live alone and have carers a few times per week.

MSE	Description
Appearance and Behaviour	You look dishevelled, your hair is messy, you have a beard. During the interview you generally appear quite fidgety and restless. When you are questioned by the candidate you occasionally appear distracted and look off into another side of the room. This is because you saw one of the children run by.
Speech	Your speech is normal in rate, volume and tone.
Mood	You sometimes feel low in mood and you have felt very lonely since your wife died two years ago. You still enjoy seeing your children and grandchildren, but they don't visit very often. You don't have many interests but you still like to watch sport on TV. Sometimes when you feel low you wonder whether life is still worth living, but you never have thoughts of killing yourself. You think that 'life is too precious.'
Thought	Thought process – the answers you give are relevant. You don't veer off topic. No one is interfering with your thoughts. Thought content – You claim that the reason you left your house was because you were frightened by the small children running around at the end of your bed. The police then kidnapped you. You could see about 3 children aged around 3 to 5 running in circles, but they did not say anything to you. You also felt unsafe in your house because you think the walls have been 'bugged'. You think they are fitted with cameras and microphones, but you don't know who did this.

	You didn't want to call your daughter because you thought people might listen to the phone call and so you decided to walk to her house but soon got lost. You haven't seen the children before, but you did see a small train passing through your living room a few days ago. You also mention that you have heard a man's voice talking about you from outside your bedroom window. You don't know who he is. You seem quite suspicious of the doctor and at one point you say "Why are you asking me all these questions? Are you from the Police?" You have strong religious beliefs based in Islam, no convictions.
Perception	You are distracted by the children running around the room.
Cognition	The year is 1982. You don't know what day, month or season it is. You think that are in a hospital or a hotel.
Insight	You admit that your memory is not as good as it once was and think that "maybe there's something wrong with my head". However, you insist that the children were real. You accept that this is strange but think that they must have accidently walked into the wrong house.
Risk	You do not have any thoughts of hurting yourself or anyone else. You don't think you would do anything to put yourself in danger because "there is nothing wrong with me."

Markscheme

Task:	Achieved	Not Achieved
Introduces self		
Clarifies who they are speaking to and gains consent from patient		
Establishes rapport		
Elicits history of recent behaviours in a concise and fluent manner		
Comments on Appearance (height, overweight/underweight, clothing, kempt/unkempt).		
Comments on Behaviour (distraction, fidgety, suspicious)		
Comments on Speech (rate/volume/tone)		
Comments on Objective Mood (low/Euthymic/Elated)		
Comments on Affect (reactive/Flat/Blunted)		
Comments on Subjective Mood (E.g. Sad, suicidal, Hopeless, Happy, Optimistic).		
Enquires specifically about suicidal thoughts and risk		
Comments on Thought Form (No disorder of thought form)		
Comments on Thought Content (Elicits paranoid thoughts/delusions, memory problems, wandering behaviour).		
Comments on Visual hallucinations (What they have seen)		
Comments on Auditory hallucinations (E.g. Who the voices are, whether they are 1st, 2nd or 3rd person, what they are saying etc.)		
Comments on cognition (Includes whether patient is orientated in time, place, and person)		
Comments on level of insight "do you think you are unwell?" "Do you think you need medication?"		

QUESTION: Performs a detailed risk assessment (including self-harm, suicide, harming others, sexual vulnerability, financial vulnerability)		
QUESTION: Provides diagnosis and suitable differential - must include dementia and delirium, others include drug induced psychosis, late-onset schizophrenia.		
Non-judgmental approach		
Examiner's Global Mark	/5	
Actor / Helper's Global Mark	/5	
Total Station Mark	/30	

Learning Points

- In a case of an acute confusional state in the old age psychiatry setting it is important to rule out delirium. The onset of symptoms is unclear and it is possible that the paranoia and hallucinations may be secondary to an infection.

- The features that differentiate delirium from other possible causes such as dementia are listed below:

- Delirium has a typical onset of hours/days, whereas symptoms of dementia commonly develop over weeks/months.
- In delirium there is typically significant fluctuation in the level of confusion throughout the day, whereas dementia usually follows a much more subtle deterioration.
- Dementia can often present with psychotic symptoms such as visual hallucinations. Hallucinations of things such as small children are particularly common in Lewy Body Dementia.

2.6 "Loneliness"

Candidate Instructions

You are the foundation year doctor reviewing an 80-year-old retired nurse called Audrey as part of your attachment to an old-age community mental health team (CMHT). The patient is well known to the CMHT and has a routine appointment in clinic.

Please take a history. You have 6 minutes to do so, after which you will be asked for a summary, risk assessment, and plan.

Examiner's Instructions

An 80-year-old returned nurse called Audrey has attended a clinic for a routine appointment with the community mental health team. The foundation year doctor has been asked to review the patient, take a history, and then summarise their findings with a risk assessment and plan.

Please stop the candidate after 6 minutes and ask for their summary, risk assessment and plan. Please prompt them to explain the reasoning behind their risk assessment.

Actor's Instructions

Background:
You are an 80-year-old retired nurse called Audrey. You have a history of recurrent depressive disorder. You have been visiting the community mental health team for the past two years since the death of your spouse which you took very badly. For the past two months your mood has become especially low.

History of symptoms:
You recently fell out with your son due an argument with your daughter-in-law. You haven't spoken for two months. He is your only child and you now feel very isolated. You feel chronically low, but especially so in the evenings. To try and manage this you started to drink before you go to bed. The drinking has escalated and you now consume about 5 cans of strong lager each day. You have tried to cut down but haven't been successful. Sometimes you have a drink first thing in the morning too.

You've started to think that there's no point in living any longer and have thought about how you might end it all. Your spouse used to take Amitriptyline for pain, and there's still a big box of tablets in your bathroom. You have finalised your will, closed your bank accounts, and written a note in case things get too much. Your plan is to eventually take all of the tablets with a bottle of vodka when you're unlikely to be disturbed. You can't see how you can possibly resolve your differences with your son and don't think things will ever get better. You feel very guilty about this.

You used to enjoy listening to the radio and reading, but now you don't have motivation for anything and feel "empty". You have poor appetite and get by on the occasional ready-meal. You have poor sleep and often wake early in the morning.

You were admitted to hospital for depression once, 20 years ago. At the time you had been made redundant and you attempted suicide by hanging, but were saved by your husband. You had a long admission for six months and after failing to respond to medication you eventually needed several sessions of ECT. Since then you've intermittently seen psychiatrists. You initially took a tablet called Citalopram which was quite effective, but had to stop 5 years ago after you developed low sodium levels. You now take a tablet called Mirtazapine but it doesn't seem to be help much.

You have a bad back and suffer from chronic pain. Aside from that your only medical problems are high blood pressure and high cholesterol. You take tablets for these but can't remember what they're called. You have no allergies.

You live alone in a two bed flat. You are fully independent. You don't smoke and have never taken recreational drugs. There is a strong family history of depression on your mother's side of the family.

Your behaviour:
Your posture is stooped, your gaze is downcast, your eye contact is poor. Your speech is slow in rate, low in volume, and monotone. You are tearful and hopeless in manner. You have no hallucinations or delusions. You are willing to seek help however, and come into hospital if needed.

Mark Scheme – "Loneliness"

Task:	Achieved	Not Achieved
Introduces self		
Clarifies who they are speaking to and obtains consent		
Establishes rapport		
Elicits history of low mood (nature, onset, timing, triggers, exacerbating factors)		
Asks specifically about self-harm and suicidal thoughts		
Ask specifically about plan		
Asks specifically about preparation (note / will / finances / attempts to avoid discovery)		
Asks about feelings of hopelessness		
Asks about anhedonia (inability to feel pleasure in normally pleasurable activities).		
Asks about psychotic symptoms (delusions or hallucinations)		
Asks about biological symptoms of low mood (sleep, appetite, weight loss, libido)		
Asks about alcohol and drug use		
Asks about past psychiatric history		
Asks about past medical history		
Asks about medications and allergies		
Asks about family history		
Asks about social history (support, accommodation, personal and domestic activities of daily living)		
Summarises case concisely		

Provides a risk assessment – considers the patient to be high risk and explains why (must include one of the following: age, alcohol use, chronic pain, active suicidality/plan).		
Provides a plan – must include some form of escalation (E.g. discuss with consultant, arrange for admission etc.)		
Examiner's Global Mark	/5	
Actor / Helper's Global Mark	/5	
Total Station Mark	/30	

Learning Points

- Depression is common in the elderly, and old age in itself is a risk factor for suicide. In such cases, it is important to always discuss your management plan with a senior.

- A useful scheme to take a history of suicidal attempt or intent is to ask about before (planning, intentions, impulsivity, will, suicide note), during (location, measures to prevent being found, method of choice) and after (regret, remorse, future plans)

- There is no evidence to suggest that discussing suicide increases the level of risk, so if you suspect that someone might be feeling suicidal then do not be afraid to ask. It is important to probe and determine the level of risk by asking about plans, notes, past attempts etc.

Child & Adolescent Mental Health (CAMHS)

3.1 "Disruptive Donny"

Candidate's Instructions:

A 12-year-old boy called Donny has presented to the GP accompanied by his mother. His teachers are concerned over frequent absences from school and that his behaviour is becoming increasingly disruptive.

You are the foundation doctor working in an inner-city GP surgery. The GP summary states he has a background of autism.

You have 7 minutes to take a history, followed by an opportunity for you to present your findings and answer a series of questions.

Examiner's Instructions:

A 12-year-old boy called Donny has come to the GP practice with his mother. His school are concerned over an increasing number of absences from school and disruptive behaviour in the classroom.

The foundation doctor at the GP surgery has been asked to take a history from the patient and mother. The GP summary states he has a background of autism.

At 7 minutes please stop the candidate and ask them to present their history and formulate an initial management plan.

Actor's Instructions:

Background
You are "at the end of your tether" with your 12-year-old son, Donny. You cannot control him and don't know what to do. You know that he has been skipping school to hang out with a crowd of older boys; they are a bad influence but you cannot keep him away from them. You had a meeting at the school, they told you that Donny has been disturbing classes, shouting verbal abuse at teachers and is struggling academically with 'F's' in his recent progress tests.

History of symptoms
You have seen Donny with these older boys around the neighbourhood smoking cannabis and drinking alcohol. You are worried that he is being pressurised into these behaviours. You have tried to keep him away from them but he gets aggressive when told to stay at home. He often gets angry by shouting and swearing at directly at you, but has never been physically violent.

He was brought home by the police last night for trying to set fire to a bus shelter. You think he often sneaks out after you have gone to sleep in the evening as his windowsill has dirty footprints on it. This was the second time he has been in trouble with the police; a month ago he stole and attacked your neighbour's dog. Donny did not show any sign of guilt, and didn't understand why he was in trouble for doing these things.

You have noticed his behaviour has been getting worse since his father left two years ago. He was having an affair and suddenly moved to another city many miles away in the space of two weeks. Donny was very close to his father, but he rarely visits anymore after the birth of Donny's step-brother Steve 6 months ago. When Donny is at home he spends most of his time in his room playing video games, if asked – he likes shooting and war games.

Donny has autism, which was diagnosed when he was 6 years old as he was not socializing with other children, and was having difficulties at school. You had a normal pregnancy; Donny was slow to start speaking but achieved all of his milestones. His primary school teachers noticed that he was slow at reading and writing compared to the other children. You tried to get him into the local school for autism but he was not accepted, as it was full. He is currently in a mainstream school and is struggling with work. You know he is a bright boy deep down, but thinks he needs more support. He does not have many friends in his year; the teachers say that he is isolated from the other school children.

He does not have any significant past medical history and outright denies drinking, smoking or taking illicit substances. However, he has come home smelling of cannabis before, and shrugs and goes quiet when this is questioned. His mother is currently being treated for depression and is unemployed. Donny lives with his mum in a small two bedroom ground floor flat in a rough housing estate and often go to the local food bank to make ends meet.

Conduct disorder STATION OSCE – "Disruptive Donny"

Task:	Achieved	Not Achieved
Introduces self		
Confirms patient identify and gain consent		
Elicits history from patient in a concise manner		
Asks about presenting complaint with an open question		
Asks about behaviour at school and at home		
Asks about interaction and relationships with other students and teachers – isolation, bullying, disruptive behaviour		
Elicits drug and alcohol use		
Asks about aggressive or destructive behaviour		
Ascertains forensic history		
Asks about feelings of guilt, regret, remorse, saying sorry		
Asks about family dynamics and situation at home		
Asks about development – motor delay, language delay and social delay		
Asks about past medical history		
Asks about past psychiatric history		
Ask about family history including familial psychiatric history		
Non judgmental approach		
Empathetic manner		
Summarises the history fluently		

Structured management plan		
Investigations to rule out organic cause – Baseline bloods including TFT, urine drug screen		
Conservative therapies – CBT, psychotherapy, anger management, impulse control, functional family therapy and parent management training, involve social worker		
Examiner's Global Mark	/5	
Actor / Helper's Global Mark	/5	
Total Station Mark	/30	

Learning Points

- Toddlers and adolescents are entitled to their challenging moments. However, if their behaviour is out of the ordinary and seriously challenges social boundaries, a disruptive behaviour disorder, such as conduct disorder (CD) or oppositional defiant disorder (ODD), can be considered.

- Both ODD and CD are characterised by a combination of antisocial behaviours violence, destroying property, substance misuse and violation of rules (theft, abuse, graffiti, arson, violence). CD usually presents in teenagers, whilst ODD presents before the age of 8. In ODD, behaviours rebellious behaviour is fixated against figures of authority.

- In the history of presenting complaint try to ascertain whether the behaviours are present at school, in the home and in social situations.

3.2 "Grace's overdose"

Candidate's Instructions:

You are a foundation doctor working in a busy emergency department. 15-year-old Grace has been brought to see you by her mother. Grace's mother found her crying next to an empty packet of paracetamol and an empty bottle of wine half an hour ago, so took her immediately to the emergency department. She has now admitted to taking the tablets.

Grace's mother has left to answer an urgent phone call and will not be present during the consultation.

Please take a history from the patient. You will be stopped after 7 minutes and asked to summarise and suggest a management plan.

Examiner's Instructions:

The candidate has been asked to take a history from 15-year-old Grace who took an overdose of paracetamol this evening and has been brought to the emergency department department by her mother.

Grace's mother has gone off to answer a phone call and will not be present during the consultation.

This station will test the candidate's history taking skills and their ability to evaluate suicide/self harm risk.

Please stop the candidate after 7 minutes and ask them to summarise their history, suggest a suicide risk category and formulate a management plan.

If the candidate mentions taking paracetamol levels in their management plan ask them when they should be taken.

State that the "levels have come back above the treatment line" and ask them how would this affect management?

Actor's Instructions:

Background
You are a 15-year-old girl called Grace who is currently studying for your GCSEs. Your Mum has taken you to the emergency department after she found you crying in your room next to an empty packet of paracetamol.

Over the last few weeks there have been a few things that have made you upset and angry. You and your boyfriend have been arguing and on two separate occasions he's called you a "fat bitch" and "not worth it". Because of this you are constantly worrying that he's going to break up with you. On top of this you are getting behind with your homework and recently underachieved in your mock GCSEs. Your Mum is putting a huge amount of pressure on you to do well in your exams and it's making you feel like a failure.

Two hours ago, in the spur of the moment, you took 18 paracetamol tablets from the bathroom cupboard and drank half a bottle of wine you found in the fridge to "make it all go away". You didn't think this would end your life and you did not write a suicide note. You immediately regretted it and text your boyfriend what had happened, hoping it would make him feel guilty. Your mum was in the next room but didn't hear you at the time. You left the wine bottle and the packet of tablets next to you rather than trying to hide them. You have never done anything like this before but feel you have been pushed into feeling this way, and that "everything is getting too much". In the past few weeks you have thought about harming yourself in some way to make your problems go away but have not acted on these thoughts. You wouldn't want to end your life because you have great family and friends and you're looking forward to going to college next year.

You enjoy shopping with your friends, spending time with your boyfriend and going to school, most of the time. You have no problems sleeping, no weight loss and your appetite is normal. You sometimes smoke cannabis with your friends and rarely drink alcohol. You have two older brothers (John 18, Paul 22) who are both at university. A few weekends ago, you went to stay with John to experience university life; you got very drunk and took a drug that all of his friends were doing called 'Black Mamba'. It made you feel psychedelic and like you saw neon coloured flowers and animals all night.

You have never been in trouble with the police. You have no known medical problems, and don't take any regular medications or have any drug allergies. You are not known to the mental health services, and there is no family history of mental illness. You don't think that you're depressed and don't want any further treatment. You are really embarrassed about what happened. You deny self-harm or suicidal ideation, and are sure this won't happen again. You don't know why your mum is making such a 'big deal out of it'.

Behaviour and appearance
You are wearing your school uniform and you usually wear lots of make up. You are usually quite chatty and confident but today you are withdrawn and embarrassed by your actions so spend most of the consultation looking down at your hands fiddling with your jewellery/clothes. You aren't sure about the answer to lots of the questions so you just shrug and say 'I don't know'.

HISTORY TAKING OSCE STATION- overdose

Task:	Achieved	Not Achieved
Introduces self		
Clarifies patient identity and gains consent		
Asks open question (elicits presenting complaint)		
Elicits events precipitating overdose – preparation, planning, suicide note, triggers		
Circumstance of overdose – alone/intoxicated and when the tablets were taken (simultaneously/ staggered)		
Asks about additional alcohol or drugs used		
Elicits type of medication and number of tablets taken		
Asks about events after the overdose – regret, hid evidence, told someone		
Asks about ongoing suicidal ideation, plans, protective factors, suicide note		
Assesses mood and elicits depressive symptoms– low mood, anhedonia, fatigue		
Asks about psychiatric history		
Asks about past medical history		
Asks about medications and allergies		
Social history –family, school, relationships, social activities, home life, smoking		
Summarises consultation appropriately		
States risk of self harm/suicide as low risk		
Suggests appropriate management plan including baseline bloods (including liver function, clotting profile) and taking paracetamol levels 4 hours post ingestion.		
States if levels are above the treatment line they will need to start an N-Acetylcysteine infusion.		
Mentions referring to the Child and Adolescent Mental Health Service for assessment.		
Non-judgemental approach		
Examiner's Global Mark	/5	
Actor / Helper's Global Mark	/5	
Total Station Mark	/30	

Learning points

- Paracetamol overdose is one of the most common psychiatric presentations to the emergency department. The important factors to ask regarding the overdose are what medication, how many tablets, what dose, staggered or simultaneous overdose, and was there a delay in presentation?

- Paracetamol undergoes breakdown in the liver to a toxic metabolite called N-acetyl-p-benzoquinoneimine (NAPQI) which depletes the liver's supply of glutathione stores. NAPQI can then cause hepatic necrosis once glutathione stores reach zero. Liver failure is therefore the biggest medical concern in patient presenting with paracetamol overdose and care needs to be taken when monitoring their paracetamol levels. N-acetylcysteine (NAC) is the antidote given to anyone above the treatment line on the paracetamol treatment graph or that presents with a significant overdose: over 12 grams (24 x 500mg tablets) or >75mg/kg. NAC can produce hypersensitivity reactions so is best given by slow intravenous infusion.

- Alcoholics and those who are chronically malnourished (e.g. anorexia nervosa, cachexia) are at higher risk of liver damage due to reduced glutathione stores.

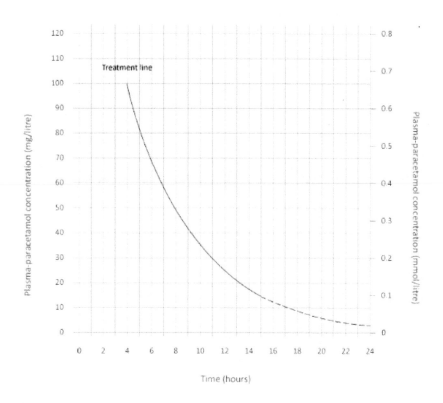

3.3 "Fussy eater"

Candidate's Instructions:

A 15-year-old girl called Olivia attends the GP surgery with her mum who booked the appointment on her behalf as she is concerned about her daughter's weight.

You are the foundation doctor based at the practice and have been asked to take a history from the patient by the principal GP. Her mother has left the room so you can talk to her daughter alone.

You have 7 minutes to take a full history after which you will be stopped and asked to present your findings and suggest an initial management plan.

Examiner's Instructions:

A 15-year-old girl called Olivia has attended the GP surgery with her mum who booked the appointment on her behalf due to concerns about her daughter's weight.

The foundation doctor based at the practice has been asked to take a history from the patient, with a view to summarising their findings and suggesting an initial management plan. Her mother has left the room so the trainee can talk to her daughter alone.

Pay particular attention to the candidate's interaction with the rather timid and defensive patient.

After 7 minutes please ask the candidate to summarise the case, and suggest an initial management plan.

Actor's Instructions:

Background
You are a 15-year-old girl called Olivia. You attend a mainstream school. Your mum has booked this appointment as she is always "going on at you" about your weight and the fact that you are a "fussy eater".

Your behaviour
You don't want to be here. You are initially introverted and quiet, and do not volunteer any information unless specifically asked. You become defensive and irritable when the topic of food is raised. However, if you feel the candidate is empathetic and non-judgemental, you gradually reveal your history.

Your history of symptoms
You had glandular fever at the age of 10, during which you had several months off school due to fatigue. During this time, you lost some weight due to illness. You began to enjoy the weight-loss, but when your weight gradually started to increase you felt fat and ugly.

You started secondary school shortly afterwards, but found it difficult to make friends. Your parents were also going through a separation at this point. You turned your attention to your studies, and achieved top grades at school. Your teachers describe you as hard-working, and a "perfectionist". You became more and more preoccupied with your weight, and began weighing yourself on a daily basis. If your weight increased, you felt fat and disgusting. You began looking on the internet for ways to lose weight, such as laxatives, heavy exercise and cutting out certain food groups. Initially you became a vegetarian, then a vegan, and today you are eating only 1 or 2 spoonfuls of low fat cereal, one spoon of low-fat yoghurt, half a protein bar and black coffee, per day. You do not binge-eat or purge.

Your mum is always "on at you" to eat more, and you have started to hide meals or throw them down the toilet in order to make her think you have eaten them. If friends invite you to their house for dinner you make excuses not to go, and as a result have few friends at school. You seldom eat in front of others. Your mum keeps telling you to eat more and says you are too thin. This causes friction between you. You try to hide your body under baggy clothes. You were learning about BMI in a lesson at school and calculated it to be 14, although when you look in the mirror you still feel overweight. Your ideal weight would be 40kg. Your periods started at the age of 12, but you have noticed that you have only had one or two periods in the last year. You feel tired all the time and find sports at school almost impossible. You have noticed that your hair is falling out quite easily.

You have no past medical history or allergies, and you do not drink alcohol or use illicit drugs. You have never thought about dying or committing suicide or seen a psychiatrist. You do not have any ritualistic or compulsive behaviours, or auditory or visual hallucinations. You are not open to treatment at this point because you are scared that you will be told to gain weight and/or be force-fed. You are happy for the information you give to be shared with your mum. You have a 21-year-old brother called Jeremy who has just finished a degree at Oxford University. There is no family history of mental illness.

ANOREXIA NERVOSA STATION OSCE – "Fussy Eater"

Task:	Achieved	Not Achieved
Introduces self and gains consent for discussion		
Clarifies patient identify and gains consent		
Asks open question to establish presenting complaint		
Asks about current eating pattern (e.g. amount, exclusion of food groups, weighing)		
Asks when symptoms first started and if there was a trigger (e.g. physical illness, abuse, bullying)		
Enquires about personality type (e.g. perfectionist, rituals, obsessions or compulsions)		
Asks about perception of body image, "what do you see in the mirror"		
Asks about weight loss behaviours: avoidance, vomiting, purging, appetite suppressants, laxatives, excessive exercise		
Asks about fear of weight gain		
Asks about current BMI, ideal weight		
Enquires about physical symptoms (e.g. amenorrhoea, fatigue, abdominal pain, fainting, delayed or arrested puberty, hair loss)		
Asks about past medical history		
Asks about past psychiatric history		
Asks about current medications and allergies		
Asks about personal history (childhood, relationships, education)		

Asks about family history, including mental health and suicide		
Asks about drug history, allergies and compliance, including comorbid drug / alcohol misuse		
Discusses impact of symptoms on life (studies, relationships)		
Summarises consultation concisely		
Explains basic steps for investigation (physical exam including calculation of BMI, bloods and ECG)		
Suggests basic management plan (encourage Olivia to speak to her mother, urgent referral to eating disorder clinic, involvement of dietician and psychological therapy)		
	/20	
Examiner's Global Mark	/5	
Actor / Helper's Global Mark	/5	
Total Station Mark	/30	

Learning Points

- Recent studies suggest that up to 25% of those with eating disorders are male. It is important to distinguish anorexia nervosa from bulimia nervosa. Both involve a distortion of body image and preoccupation with food, however bulimics are often of normal body weight, and undergo episodes of binge eating with purging.

- Admission to hospital will need to be considered when the BMI is less than 15 kg/m2 or when there are medical complications such as electrolyte disturbance, bradycardia or pronounced oedema.

- The diagnostic criteria for anorexia:
  Low body weight (<15% of expected weight) and BMI (<17.5)
  Self-induced weight loss/fear of weight gain (including excessive exercise, food restriction and laxative abuse)
  Distorted body image
  Endocrine disturbances (amenorrhoea and reduced sexual drive)
  Delayed/arrested puberty

3.4 "The Bohemian Busy Bee"

Candidate's Instructions:

You are a foundation year doctor currently on your GP placement. You have been allocated your own clinic this morning. The first patient is Mary who has come to talk to you regarding some concerns she has for her 10-year-old son called Blake.

You have 7 minutes to take a history, after which you will be asked to formulate a differential diagnosis.

Examiner's Instructions:

A 40-year-old mum called Mary has come into her GP surgery to discuss her concerns regarding her 10-year-old son named Blake.

The foundation year doctor has been asked to take a history from the mother and to formulate a differential diagnosis based on the symptoms described.

Please stop the candidate at 7 minutes and ask for their differential diagnoses, and reasoning behind their choices.

Actor's Instruction:

Background
You are a 40-year-old mother of two called Mary. You have come to discuss your youngest child Blake who is 10 years old. You are a sculptor and a free spirit. You are wearing bohemian style of clothing.

History of symptoms
You have received some worrying school reports regarding your son's academic performance. His homework is never complete and it often contains careless mistakes. Before starting class, Blake is always messing about in the playground and the teacher has to individually call him in to get class started. He forgets his homework book more times than he has it. During class, he complains that he is bored and cannot focus on the task at hand. He is often told to leave class so not to disrupt learning for others. He has been asked to move seat countless times as other mums have complained that Blake is hindering their child's learning.

The issues arose ever since he moved school at the age of 6. He was very well incorporated at his old school, 'Beehurst', which was a liberal independent school that taught through exploration and independence. Blake worked well in this environments, energetically rushing about the class finding objects and books related to the subject of the day. It was noted that he was the class finder but he did not like to sit down with the book and read it for very much time before moving on to the next object. Now that he has moved to a new school, there has been a more traditional approach to learning with homework and quiet study and it's "just not suited to Blake's predisposition". The teachers are worried that if he continues to make careless mistakes he will not do well academically.

Despite this, he is a happy and popular child. He always makes good eye contact and he is not obsessive or impulsive. He has never reported hearing or seeing anything that was not there. He once was involved in a school fight but he told you he had not started it. He has been aggressive to his sister in the normal sibling sort of way, fighting over the laptop. He is a bohemian busy bee at home working on his sculpting with you. He loves to make a mess.

He has no history of depression, anxiety or schizophrenia. When asked about family history, your other child, Octavia, is a healthy 12-year-old that is well integrated socially and academically at the same school. Blake was induced 2 weeks early because there were concerns about his movement levels, but was thankfully born a happy and healthy baby.

Your husband was expelled from secondary school for serious prank in which he called the police claiming there was a bomb threat in the girls' loos. Now you think of it, your husband does hate to be stuck watching the theatre. Could this mean he has something wrong with him, and is it all your fault?!

ADHD HISTORY STATION OSCE - The Bohemian Busy Bee

Task:	Achieved	Not Achieved
Introduces self		
Clarifies who they are speaking to and relationship to child and gains consent		
Elicits history from parent in a concise manner		
Establishes symptoms came on at 6 years of age		
Establishes symptoms of inattention (e.g. making careless mistakes in homework, forgetting his book, not sitting down to read a book for long, becoming bored in class)		
Establishes symptoms of hyperactivity: (e.g. needing to be called in from the playground, being disruptive during class, energetically finding books).		
Asks about symptoms of impulsivity (e.g. has he been aggressive, does he misbehave by speaking out and does he act out of turn not considering the consequences).		
Asks about function at school		
Asks about function with friends and forming relationships		
Asks about behaviour at home		
Asks about past medical history and regular medications or allergies		
Asks about past psychiatric history		
Asks about brief birth history and developmental milestones		
Asks about symptoms of autistic spectrum disorder		

Rules out depression and anxiety symptoms		
Asks about family history		
Finds out ideas, concerns and expectations		
States differential diagnosis - ADHD, OCD, Conduct disorder, hearing or visual disability,		
Gives clear explanation as to why ADHD is the most likely (age of onset, symptoms, family history, poor function at school).		
Non-judgmental approach		
Examiner's Global Mark	/5	
Actor / Helper's Global Mark	/5	
Total Station Mark	/30	

Learning Points

- ADHD is common with 2.4% of children having the developmental disorder and is four times commoner in males.[2]

- The DSM IV outlines three main subtypes:

  - Predominantly inattentive (ADD)
  - Predominantly hyperactive-impulsive subtype
  - Combined subtype (ADHD)

- Parents need a great deal of support when their children are diagnosed with ADHD. Often they experience guilt and worry that they're to blame. Some parents may feel relief that they finally have a diagnosis and it allows for optimisation of parental techniques in order to suit the child's needs. There are a huge number of ADHD support groups that parents can be put in touch with (e.g. ADDISS. AADD-UK)

- If symptoms persist, children should be referred to CAMHS for a formal assessment and diagnosis of ADHD. At this stage drug treatment may be considered. Treatment includes psycho-education, behavioural interventions, school interventions and medication in moderate to severe cases. Current medications licensed for ADHD include Methylphenidate (Ritalin), Atomoxetine and Dexamfetamine and should not be started at primary care.

3.5 "Cheeky Charlie and his Yummy Mummy"

Candidate's Instructions:

A 32-year-old stay-at-home mum has come into the GP surgery to discuss her 5-year-old son Charlie. He has been a bit cheeky and troublesome of late and she has presented with the hope of getting a prescription of Ritalin to help him concentrate. The GP has assessed Charlie on a number of occasions and felt he does not meet the criteria for ADHD.

You are and foundation doctor based at the GP practice and you have been asked to take a brief history and discuss Ritalin treatment with the mother.

You have 7 minutes for your discussion after which you will be asked to summarize your discussion to the patient.

Examiner's Instructions:

A 32-year-old stay-at-home mum has come into the GP surgery to discuss her 7-year-old son Charlie. He has been a bit cheeky and troublesome of late and she has presented with the hope of getting a prescription of Ritalin to help him concentrate. The GP has assessed Charlie on a number of occasions and not felt he meets the criteria for ADHD.

The candidate is a Foundation doctor based at the GP practice and has been asked to take a brief history and discuss Ritalin treatment with the mother.

At 7 minutes please ask the candidate to summarize the discussion to the patient.

Actor's Instructions:

Background
You are a well-kempt 32-year-old 'stay-at-home' mum who has come into the GP surgery to discuss your 7-year-old son Charlie. He's been a bit cheeky and troublesome of late and you were reading on an internet forum for worried mums called 'MumsNet' that a medication called Ritalin might help him get better grades at school.

Your behaviour
You are organized and well mannered. You have a pen and paper on you and bullet point everything that is said in the consultation. You are keen to know more about the drug and what is best for your son. You interpret often and ask lots of questions.

Your history of symptoms
Charlie, your only child, has been getting a little cheeky as he has grown older. He runs around outside and plays in the grass and shouts and screams in the playground. He sometimes forgets to put his toys away when asked to and doesn't always do as he is told. You are worried he might have a pre-occupation with food as there has been the odd occasion where he has refused to eat all his vegetables- one episode was so bad that he began crying and you were forced to give in. You are doing all you can to help Charlie learn and develop into a clever, kind and healthy young man. Sometime this just doesn't go to plan and he just doesn't want to listen to you even when you try your best.

You were doing some research online and came across an interesting post on an internet forum for mums about how a scatty young boy was transformed by taking a drug called 'Ritalin.' You have also read articles online explaining that it could help children concentrate so that they can get better grades at school. You were hoping to start this early to give little Charlie the head start he needs before the other mother's start giving it to their children.

You know that Charlie is a clever boy, he is your son of course! But he has also had glowing reports from his teachers and recently won an award for top class reader. You want him to achieve more in maths class however, as this has never been his strong point. He is the middle set at school and you know he can do better as his father is a university maths lecturer.

Charlie is otherwise fit and well, takes no medications and has no drug allergies. You had bulimia as a teenager but have no current mental health issues, and neither do the rest of your family. Charlie was born at full term by planned Caesarean section and there have been no developmental concerns.

Expectations

You are curious about the drug and wonder whether it would work for your son by improving his concentration and potential. Your husband thinks that you are too concerned about little Charlie and you compromised on this disagreement by agreeing you would discuss it with your GP to get further advice.

Ritalin counselling OSCE STATION – Cheeky Charlie and his Yummy Mummy

Task:	Achieved	Not Achieved
Introduces self		
Clarifies who they are speaking to and gains consent		
Establishes nature of Charlie's behaviour (features, onset, duration, triggers, timing, setting)		
Asks about hyperactivity (e.g. inability to sleep)		
Asks about inattention (e.g. not completing tasks)		
Asks about impulsivity (e.g. running in front of traffic)		
Establishes mother's current knowledge about Ritalin		
Establishes how much/what specifically the mother wants to know about Ritalin		
Explains that Ritalin is a stimulant drug licensed for use in ADHD in children >6 years old		
Explains benefits of using Ritalin: it can control difficult behaviours by increasing concentration and reducing impulsivity.		
Explains side effects of using Ritalin including abdominal pain, nausea, decreased appetite, insomnia, tics, autonomic side effects- dry mouth		
Investigations before treatment (blood pressure, height and weight, liver function tests)		
Ritalin requires regular monitoring (height every 6 months, weight every 6 months, heart rate and blood pressure every 3 months)		
Mentions that Ritalin use requires drug holidays due to the dangers of long term use and growth suppression		
Summarises discussion appropriately avoiding jargon		
Reassures mother that Charlie is likely going through normal development and has no concerning features.		
Explains that ADHD is diagnosed based on a comprehensive assessment involving a specialist paediatrician or psychiatrist. Charlie is not		

exhibiting any of the criteria and will therefore not benefit from assessment		
Advises against Ritalin for Charlie for the moment		
Offers leaflets and/or directs mother to appropriate resources for further information		
Allows the patient's mum to express her thoughts and concerns		
Examiner's Global Mark	/5	
Actor / Helper's Global Mark	/5	
Total Station Mark	/30	

Learning Points

- This is a hard station. Take it a step at a time and talk through the mother's concerns, in-depth details of the side-effects and mechanism of action of Ritalin are not needed here. That's specialist stuff. This type of station can be alarming, but don't be fooled, all you need is some good communication skills and an awareness of the limitations of your knowledge. Offer leaflets and other patient resources to help.

- A basic understanding of Ritalin (the trade name for methylphenidate) is enough to suffice here. It is a CNS stimulant which seems counterintuitive as children are already "fully of energy." It works by stimulating areas of the brain which aid concentration, however, can also cause nervousness, depression, irritability, drowsiness, GI upset, growth depression and suicidal ideation amongst many other side effects. Patients can also become tolerant of and dependent on this drug.

- Always put the patient first – do not let relatives influence what is best for the child. Be open, honest and reassure the mother that Charlie is developing well and is clearly already a high achiever at school. Explain he is unlikely to benefit from the medication in this case so the risks out-weigh the pros.

3.6 "Cut deep"

Candidate's Instructions:

You are a foundation year doctor working in the emergency department. A 15-year-old girl called Natalia has attended with a deep laceration on her forearm. The ED nurse practitioner has sutured the wound. The patient has revealed that it is self-inflicted, and the nurse asks you to speak to her.

Please take a history from the patient about her history of self-harm and current risk status. You have 5 minutes to complete the history, after which the examiner will stop you to ask some further questions.

Examiner's Instructions:

A foundation year doctor is working in a busy eemrgency department. They are asked to see a 15-year-old called Natalia, who self-harmed. The doctor is asked to take a history of her self-harm and to establish her current risk.

Emphasis should be placed on the candidate's ability to ask potentially difficult questions sensitively and to behave professionally and compassionately towards the patient.

They should also clearly distinguish deliberate self-harm from attempted suicide in the risk assessment.

Please stop the candidate at 5 minutes, so that you can ask some further questions:

1.   QUESTION: What do you consider the risk to be?
Prompt the candidate to describe the risk to self and to others.

2.   QUESTION: Now that she has spoken to you she feels ready to be discharged from A&E and is planning to go home. What options would you consider in your management plan?

3.   QUESTION: Who else would you speak to?

Actor's Instructions:

Background:
You are a 15-year-old young girl called Natalia who has come to the emergency department with a deep cut on your forearm, which was self-inflicted. The foundation year doctor has been asked to come and speak to you in more detail about it. You cut yourself today after a row with your mother. You were very angry and did it impulsively. You didn't intend to cut yourself deeply and had no wish to end your life or attend hospital. You suffer from depression and mood swings, and you are known to a Children and Adolescent Mental Health Service (CAMHS). You have regular meetings with your care coordinator, who you are due to see next week.

History of symptoms:
You always cut yourself superficially on your arms and legs, and you have never self-harmed by any other means. This is the first time you have ever cut yourself deeply enough to require any intervention or attendance to ED.

You have been cutting yourself on and off since the age of 12. You can't remember why or how you started, but you find it helps when you are feeling distressed or out of control. It provides momentary relief. You usually cut yourself at least once a week and this has not changed recently. You also used to bang your head repeatedly on the wall until you got a bruise but you haven't done this for a few years. You have never blacked out.

You have no medical conditions and do not take any regular medication. You live with your parents, who are both teachers, and you have a boyfriend who is supportive. You attend a mainstream school which is going well. You see the school counselor occasionally when you feel stressed. Your parents know about your mental health problems and one of them accompanies you to your appointments with the CAMHS team and your social worker. They know about your cutting and your Mother came with you to A&E

today. No-one else in your family has any history of mental health problems or self-harm. You do not use any drugs but you do binge-drink at the weekends when you are with friends. You do not drink alone. You were born at full term and there have been no developmental concerns (walking and talking at all the normal times).

Your behaviour:
You are rational and not distressed; you have calmed down after the altercation with your mother. You feel embarrassed. You have no plans to cut or hurt yourself now or in the immediate future, although you acknowledge that you will continue to cut yourself superficially as a form of relief. You do not feel severely depressed. You have never experienced any delusional or paranoid beliefs, and you have never heard voices or seen things that aren't there. You would like to go home. You do not want to come into hospital.

Psych OSCE – Deliberate Self-Harm History

Task:	Achieved	Not Achieved
Introduces self to patient		
Clarifies who they are speaking to and obtains consent		
Establishes rapport		
Elicits history of symptoms (nature, onset, timing, exacerbating factors)		
Establishes trigger for DSH (row with mother)		
Establishes severity / intent: did not intend to end her life		
Asks about core symptoms of depression (low mood, anhedonia, fatigue)		
Asks about psychotic symptoms		
Asks about past psychiatric history		
Asks about past medical history, medication and allergies		
Enquires about drug and alcohol use		
Asks about social history (alcohol, smoking, childhood)		
Asks about personal history (childhood, relationships, school, brief birth and developmental history)		
Asks about family history (mental illness, suicide)		
Risk assessment: asks about current suicidal ideation, likelihood to self-harm		
Risk assessment: asks about other risk factors; e.g. risk to others or from others.		
Question: What do you consider the risk to be? Factors to consider (nature of attempt – i.e. impulsive, no current suicidal ideation, social support (parents/ boyfriend), alcohol use – increased risk, age places her in higher risk category.)		
Question: What options would you consider in your management plan? Offering an informal admission, or discharging with follow-up from the community team or crisis team involvement, telephone or home visit. Discharge would be considered if family or friends would be able to stay with her and keep		

an eye on her. Advising to see GP for follow up in next few days.		
Question: Who else would you speak to? Parents, patient's mental health team if available, care coordinator, or liaison team if out of hours.		
Non-judgmental approach		
Examiner's Global Mark	/5	
Actor / Helper's Global Mark	/5	
Total Station Mark	/30	

Learning Points

- "Self-harm" covers a broad range of behaviours. Cutting is the commonest form seen in adolescents in the community, whilst in inpatient units self-poisoning (e.g. paracetamol overdose) is commoner. *Remember that self-harm can be with or without suicidal intent.*

- 10% of adolescents report having self-harmed, but only about 1 in 8 of these will present to services. It is therefore particularly important for healthcare professionals to talk to young people about the issues of self-harm and suicide.

Some key risk factors for **suicide** in adolescents are:

- Male gender (although females are more likely to self-harm - particularly between the ages of 12 and 15, when the female-to-male ratio is approximately 5:1)
- Family history of suicide
- Lower socioeconomic status
- Parental separation, divorce or death
- A co-existing mental disorder – particularly depression, anxiety and ADHD
- Alcohol and drug misuse

3.7 "Cybersadness"

Candidate's Instructions:

You are a foundation year doctor currently on your CAMHS placement. You are asked by your consultant to see your own patients this morning. The first patient is a 16-year-old girl called Sam.

Please take a focused history. You will be stopped after 6 minutes to provide a diagnosis.

Examiner's Instructions:

A 16-old girl called Sam has been referred to CAMHS by her GP. The foundation year doctor has been asked to take a focused history from her and to formulate a diagnosis based on the symptoms described.

Please stop the candidate at 6 minutes and ask them to state the diagnoses and discuss potential triggers for this.

1. QUESTION: What is your diagnosis?
2. QUESTION: How would you grade the severity, and why? (Mild, moderate or severe)

Actor's Instructions:

Background:
You are a 16-year-old schoolgirl called Sam who has been referred to see a child and adolescent psychiatrist by your GP.

Behaviour:
You are looking down toward your feet at the start of the interview. You are shy and have crossed your arms on your lap. You didn't want to come and see a psychiatrist and you feel worried about making things worse. Initially speak quietly and timidly, looking at the ground. As the foundation doctor makes you feel at ease start speaking more loudly and coherently. You should look sad and may be tearful at times when speaking about the difficulties you have encountered.

History of symptoms:
For the past four months you have been bullied at school by a group of 4 girls who you used to be friends with. You are larger than the other girls and it started with name-calling such as "fatty, piggy, supersize". This has escalated and now they are writing horrible messages on your social media page. Recently someone hacked into your social media account and wrote a message on your timeline saying "I am such an unhappy slut. I might as well kill myself". Over 40 people liked this before you managed to take it down. They have created an online page called "We hate Sam" and over a 100 people have joined. At school other students have started ignoring you and laughing behind your back. You have no friends. So far the bullying has been psychological only. But the bullies have threatened to hurt you physically if you tell anyone. You haven't reported any of this to anyone and you wish the situation would just "go away". You have started skipping school to avoid the bullying, which is why your mum made you see the GP, but the online bullying means you can never escape. You are not sure if you are depressed but you would like help to feel "back to normal".

You do not have suicidal thoughts and you would never to do anything to hurt yourself. You have clear thoughts for the future including wanting to become a painter one day. You do not have psychotic symptoms. You do not have any medical problems, regular medications or allergies. You do not smoke, drink alcohol, or take drugs. You were born at full term and there were no developmental concerns (walking and talking at the normal times). You attend mainstream school. Your parents divorced when you were 7 and you now live with your mother, step-father and their new 9-month old baby. Home has been busy with the new baby. You see your biological father every other weekend. You describe a happy childhood, despite your parent's divorce. You are not known to the child and adolescent mental health services, or social services. No family history of mental illness or suicide.

Mental state:
As a result of the bullying you have started feeling low all day every day for the past three months. Your mood is at its lowest when you are about to go to school. Whilst you still enjoy watching TV, reading books, painting and being with your family, you feel tired all the time. You have disturbed sleep and find that you are waking up at 4am every day. You have been overeating, as food has become your only comfort and friend. Your concentration has become poor and your grades at school are getting worse. Your self confidence is rock bottom and you feel the situation is hopeless. You do not feel guilty as you recognize that the bullying isn't your fault.

BULLYING STATION OSCE - Cyberbullying

Task:	Achieved	Not Achieved
Introduces self		
Clarifies patient identify and obtains consent		
Elicits history of symptoms a concise and logical manner		
Establishes nature of the bullying (onset, triggers, timing, duration, exacerbating factors)		
Establishes severity of bullying		
Establishes core symptoms of depression (low mood, anhedonia, fatigue)		
Asks about *at least three* biological symptoms of depression (diurnal variations in mood, appetite and weight loss, disturbed sleep including early morning waking, reduced libido)		
Asks about *at least two* other symptoms of depression (guilt, hopelessness, poor concentration or indecisiveness, low self-confidence, agitation or slowing of movement)		
Asks about symptoms of anxiety		
Asks about previous episodes of low mood		
Asks about any previous episodes of mania		
Asks about psychotic symptoms		
Asks about self harm or suicidal thoughts		
Asks about past psychiatric history		
Asks about past medical history, medications and allergies		
Asks about family history		

Asks about social history (alcohol, smoking, drugs, occupation)		
Asks about personal history (childhood, relationships, school, brief birth and developmental history)		
Provides appropriate diagnosis, including severity (depression, mild-moderate)		
Gives clear explanation as to why mild-moderate depression (duration, symptoms)		
Examiner's Global Mark	/5	
Actor / Helper's Global Mark	/5	
Total Station Mark	/30	

Learning Points

- Bullying is defined as repeated behaviour that is intended to hurt someone either physically or emotionally. There are many different types of bulling including:

Verbal- e.g.- name calling, teasing and threats
Physical bullying- e.g.- hair pulling, hitting, pushing
Social bullying- e.g.- social excluding people, spreading rumours
Cyberbullying- any bullying that involves the use of digital technology such as phone harassment, abusive messages, writing rude comments on social media, imitating others online

- Supporting young people with low mood who are the victims of bullying can be thought of at the individual, class, and school level:

Individual level- the bullying should be reported and serious discussions should be help with bullies and the victim. Role-play and group therapy have been shown to be helpful.
Class level –The class rules should include a clear message that bullying won't be tolerated and a curriculum that promotes kindness and conflict resolution
School- bullying awareness week, regular education sessions for staff, increased supervision in playground and cafeterias, ongoing meetings between parents and staff, a central group of psychologists, counsellors, school nurses who are responsible for the antibullying programme

- If there is no response and they are suffering with moderate to severe depression a multidisciplinary review is required before offering a trial of fluoxetine. Any children or young person started on fluoxetine should be reviewed closely for suicidal behaviour, self-harm or hostility.

3.8 "Poop problems"

Candidate's Instructions:

You are a foundation year doctor working in a GP practice. A mother has brought her 6-year-son Jack in as she is concerned that he has begun soiling himself.

Please take a history from the child's mother with a view to forming a likely diagnosis and management plan. The examiner will stop you at 5 minutes to ask you some questions,

Examiner's Instructions:

The candidate is a foundation year doctor working in a GP practice. They have been asked to take a history from a mother, whose 6-year-old son Jack has recently begun soiling himself.

Please stop the candidate at 5 minutes so that you can ask the following questions:

1. QUESTION: What do you think is the likely underlying cause of the soiling?
See mark scheme – soiling seems to coincide with a significant upheaval in the family; a new baby, parents initially spending a lot of time in hospital. This suggests it may be emotional in origin – however, physical conditions can also cause soiling and need to be ruled out.

2. QUESTION: Jack's Mother asks if his behaviour is "deliberate" and if she should be punishing him, eg by withdrawing TV. What advice would you give her?
Soiling is very rarely "deliberate"; often the child is embarrassed and upset and will actually go to lengths to conceal the problem. Regardless, it is important not to view it as bad behaviour or to respond by punishing the child, as this can exacerbate the problem.

3. QUESTION: What would you suggest as part of your management plan?
It is always good practice to rule out a physical cause, even if the history points towards a behavioural or psychological cause. A full physical examination would be appropriate, with treatment of any conditions like constipation that may be contributing. You could consider referring to a specialist team (such as paediatrics or children's mental health services) for further assessment and advice.

Actor's Instructions:

Background:
You are a mother whose 6-year-old son, Jack, has recently started soiling himself. You are very concerned, and have brought him to the GP to speak to a doctor about it.

History of symptoms:
Jack started soiling himself during the day about two months ago – initially you thought it he was just a bit unwell, but then his school rang you to say he had had an accident in the playground. It is now happening almost every day, sometimes at school. Before this he was fully toilet trained. He is not having problems at night.

You are very worried that he has "behavioural problems"; his school has called you in several times to wash and change him. He doesn't seem to be constipated – some of the time he goes to the toilet normally, and he doesn't have any abdominal pain, bleeding, vomiting, straining or other symptoms. There have been no dietary correlations or changes. He seems embarrassed and upset but isn't able to explain what is happening.

There has recently been a period of emotional upheaval at home. You have had a second child about three months ago who was very unwell and was in intensive care for a month. This meant that you and your husband were often away from home. The baby is now at home, and although you're trying to include Jack you are finding it difficult. Please don't volunteer this information immediately, but use it if the candidate enquires about any possible triggers or recent changes in the family.

If asked, you do have some other concerns about Jack's behaviour – he has become much more withdrawn and "clingy" and he has stopped wanting to go to friends' houses after school. You do not think he is being bullied.

Until recently, Jack has always been a healthy and happy child. He is not known to the child and adolescent mental health services. He does not have separation anxiety. He has had no major illnesses and no concerns have been raised. He has been attending school for over a year and doing well. He had a normal birth and reached all his developmental milestones as expected (walking by 1st birthday, speech not delayed). He does not take any medication. You work part time as a teaching assistant but are currently on maternity leave, and your partner is a cab driver. You are not known to social services.

Jack lives with you, his father and now your new baby. There are no problems at home, apart from the recent illness of Jack's new baby brother, and you and your husband are caring and supportive parents. There is no family history of mental illness.

Soiling in a child – "poop problems"

Task:	Achieved	Not Achieved
Introduces self		
Clarifies who they are speaking to and gains consent		
Establishes rapport		
Elicits history of presenting symptoms (nature, onset, timing, setting)		
Enquires about coinciding physical symptoms – e.g asks about pain, constipation, diet.		
Establishes coinciding behavioural changes – more withdrawn, less cheerful, school refusal		
Enquires about child's response to soiling – he seems ashamed but can't explain how/ why		
Asks about potential triggers – bullying, changes at home		
Asks about coexisting psychiatric symptoms – mood, delusions, rituals, obsessions, checking, washing, anxiety, hyperactivity		
Asks about past history of behavioural or emotional problems		
Asks whether known to child and adolescent mental health services		
Asks about past medical history, medications, allergies		
Asks about family history		
Asks about social history (who is at home, environment, parents occupations, social worker)		
Asks about personal history (childhood, school performance, friends, brief birth and developmental history)		
Question 1: Identifies likely emotional cause of soiling. Able to name some other possible causes e.g constipation.		
Question 2: Awareness that soiling is almost never "deliberate" and advice that punishment may make it worse.		
Question 3: Able to form a sensible plan: e.g detailed physical examination to rule out physical cause, further exploration of any other underlying		

psychological factors, consider referral to local CAMHS service or specialist nurse.		
Communicates clearly and professionally		
Empathetic manner		
Examiner's Global Mark	/5	
Actor / Helper's Global Mark	/5	
Total Station Mark	/30	

Learning Points

- Encopresis or soiling is not uncommon and can cause enormous stress to the child and their family. 1 in 30 children aged 4-5 and 1 in 50 children aged 5-6 will be affected. Most children achieve day and night bowel control between the ages of 3 and 4 – usually before bladder control.

- Causes may be developmental (such as a learning disability), biological (eg constipation and overflow incontinence), behavioural (eg fear of toilets, or over-activity) or psychological in the context of stress or trauma. Often it involves a combination of factors.

- Typically, altered toileting habits (often when starting school) can lead to constipation and pain when passing stool. A vicious cycle can ensue leading to avoidance, further build up of stool, loss of normal sensation and eventually leaking of soft stool, or overflow incontinence. In this situation the encopresis is likely to be continuous, and to occur at night as well. The DSM-IV recognizes two subtypes: with constipation and overflow incontinence (requiring laxatives and "toilet retraining"), and without constipation and overflow incontinence. The latter usually responds very well to behavioural management programmes.

Forensic Psychiatry, Ethics & Law

4.1 "HELP. They won't stay"

Candidate Instructions

You are a foundation year doctor on-call covering a psychiatric inpatient hospital. You are called by one of the nurses regarding a 45-year-old patient called Emre, who is trying to leave one of the assessment wards.

Emre initially agreed to an informal admission, but the nurse thinks that recent changes in their mental state and risk mean that they would now be unsafe to leave.

Please take a handover from the nurse in SBAR format. You have 5 minutes to do so, after which you will be asked for a summary, risk assessment, and initial plan.

Examiner's Instructions

The foundation year doctor on-call covering a psychiatric inpatient hospital, has been called by a nurse regarding a patient who wants to leave the assessment ward. The 45-year-old patient, Emre, agreed to an informal admission yesterday with hypomanic symptoms. Emre has been staying awake throughout the night and as noted to be grandiose. The patient was admitted because in the past they have been quite high-risk, with impulsive and disinhibited behaviour. Since being admitted the patient has deteriorated and they are now suffering from a manic psychosis. They want to leave the ward, but the nurse on duty does not think this is safe. The candidate has been asked to take a handover from the nurse (who knows the patient well) in SBAR format, provide a summary, risk assessment, and initial plan.

Stop the candidate after 5 minutes and ask for the summary and plan. Then ask the following questions, (answers highlighted in bold text):

1.   QUESTION: If the candidate does not mention the option of a **Section 5(2)** in their plan, please ask: What is the name of the section of the Mental Health Act (1983) that you could use in this situation, without the need for other mental health professionals?"

2.   QUESTION: Then ask, "How long is this section applicable for?" **(72 hours)**

3.   QUESTION: "What is the name of the Section that nurses can also use to detain an inpatient without the need of other health professionals?" **(Section 5(4))**

4.   QUESTION: "How long is this section applicable for?" **(6 hours)**

5.   QUESTION: "The following day, the ward consultant reviewed the patient and made a first recommendation for Section 3 as he believes Emre is suffering a relapse of his bipolar affective disorder, what other professionals are needed to complete the Mental Health Act assessment?"

(Independent doctor and an Approved Mental Health Practitioner (or social worker)).

6.   QUESTION: "How long is a Section 3 applicable for?" **(6 months)**

7.   QUESTION: "What is the defined purpose of Section 3?" **(Treatment order)**

Actor's Instructions

You are a nurse on night duty in an assessment ward in a psychiatric inpatient hospital.

Situation:
Emre is a 45-year-old informal patient who was admitted yesterday and has rapidly deteriorated. He believes he works for MI5 and wants to leave the ward so that he can "take out" the man who lives in the flat opposite as he is an informant for a terrorist organisation.

Nursing staff have tried to persuade him to go to bed and reconsider things in the morning, but he is insistent that he wants leave and is becoming increasingly agitated.

Background:
Emre was admitted yesterday with symptoms of hypomania – he had been slightly grandiose, talking very quickly about how intelligent he was, and had poor sleep. He has a background of bipolar affective disorder, and is on lithium and sodium valproate. Yesterday, his presentation was not worrying, he was low risk, and was not thought to be detainable. He agreed to an informal admission.

Emre lives in supported accommodation and so staff alerted his case to his community mental health team. His community psychiatrist recommended an admission, because in the past he has been quite high-risk. In previous episodes he has become very manic, as you remember from a previous admission. On one occasion he disappeared from his accommodation for 5 days, was arrested by Police in Scotland and needed transferring back to England. When manic he can be quite aggressive and he once assaulted a member of the public. During the last admission he was not containable on the ward and spent several days in secluded isolation on the psychiatric intensive care unit (PICU).

Assessment:
This evening he has been very hostile, pacing up and down the ward and shouting at the nursing station. He is believing he is a leading MI5 agent who has uncovered top secret information about the government, and now everyone on the ward is after him and trying to poison him to erase his memory. He has not eaten or drunk anything as he is so fixated on his task to take down the terrorist organisation.

Recommendations:
You, and the rest of the nursing staff, are quite worried about him and don't think he is safe to leave the ward.

After 6 minutes, you ask the candidate "Doctor, Emre is trying to leave the ward. What should we do?"

Mark scheme

Task:	Achieved	Not Achieved
Introduces self		
Clarifies who they are speaking to and location (nurse, inpatient ward)		
Clarifies name and DOB of patient in question		
SITUATION: Asks an open question to establish the current situation in a concise manner (nature, onset, triggers, timing, exacerbating factors)		
BACKGROUND: Asks about patients background, when admitted, progress since admission		
ASSESSMENT: Asks about assessments so far, mental health observations, mood, elation, eating and drinking, sleep		
RECOMMENDATIONS: Asks what the nurse would recommend, any de-escalation tried so far, any as required medications on patients chart		
Asks about patient's current risk to self		
Asks about patient's current risk to others		
Asks about patient's current risk from others		
Asks about past risk behaviour		
QUESTION 1: Nurse asks: Doctor, Emre is trying to leave the ward. What should we do? Section 5(2) and will come to review patient		
QUESTION 2: *How long is this section applicable for?* 72 hours		
QUESTION 3: *What is the name of the Section that nurses can also use to detain an inpatient without the need of other health professionals?* Section 5(4)		
Question 4: *How long is this section applicable for?* 6 hours		
QUESTION 5: *The following day, the ward consultant reviewed the patient and made a first recommendation for Section 3, what other professionals are needed to complete the Mental Health Act assessment?* Independent doctor and an Approved Mental Health Practitioner (or social worker)		
QUESTION 6: *How long is a Section 3 applicable for?* 6 months		

QUESTION 7: *What is the defined purpose of Section 3?* Treatment order		
Non-judgmental approach		
Remains calm throughout		
Examiner's Global Mark	/5	
Actor / Helper's Global Mark	/5	
Total Station Mark	/30	

Learning Points

- It is important to have a basic understanding of the MHA. Any fully registered doctor is qualified to perform a Section 5(2) and this can be used if a patient is thought to be suffering from "any disorder of disability of the mind" and is a risk to themselves or others. Section 5(2) is an 'emergency section' and lasts 72 hours, providing time for a mental health team to consider / arrange a formal Mental Health Act Assessment (MHAA), even if it falls on a weekend.

- The other sections that it is important to know about are Sections 2 and 3. Both of these require an assessment by an independent doctor (not directly employed by the trust providing the patient's care) and an approved mental health practitioner (AMHP). AMHPs are usually qualified social workers. Section 2 lasts up to 28 days and is for 'assessment and treatment'. Section 3 lasts up to 6 months, at which point it can be renewed for a further 6 months, and thereafter it can be renewed on a yearly basis. Section 3 must be made in the agreement of the patient's nearest relative. If the nearest relative does not agree, it is still possible to proceed with Section 3, but the disagreements between the medical team and the relative must be deliberated in court.

- When taking a handover on the phone, always try to use the SBAR (situation, background, assessment, recommendation) framework.

Brief Guide to Sections of the Mental Health Act

Section of the MHA	Who can implement it?	Purpose	Length	Comments
Section 5(2)	Any fully registered doctor	Emergency	72 Hours	This can be used to stop an informal patient from leaving a mental health ward, and can also be used to stop a patient leaving a ward in a general hospital. It should only be used in circumstances where an assessment for Section 2 or 3 is not possible (commonly out of hours).
Section 5(4)	Any qualified nurse	Emergency	6 Hours	This is rarely used, but is an option if a doctor is not available to consider for Section 5(2).
Section 2	Needs two Section 12 approved doctors * and an AMHP **	Assessment and Treatment	28 Days	This is used in patients who have not been detained before, or in those who have not been assessed for a long time.
Section 3	Needs two section 12 approved doctors, an AMHP, and approval of the nearest relative	Treatment	6 Months	This can be used in patients who are well known to services and do not need a Section 2; or in those who have been admitted under Section 2 and still need to be detained after 28 days. A form of treatment must be available for it to be valid.

Section 136	The Police	Emergency	72 Hours	This is used by the Police if they find someone in a public place who is thought to be "suffering from mental disorder" and in "immediate need of care or control". Police can then take the individual to a "Place of Safety" which is usually either a room in A&E or a "136 Suite," where they can be assessed by a doctor.

* A doctor who is 'approved' under Section 12 of the Act is approved on behalf of the Secretary of State (or the Welsh Ministers) as having special expertise in the diagnosis and treatment of 'mental disorders'. Doctors who are approved clinicians are automatically also approved under Section 12. Section 12 approved doctors have a role in deciding whether someone should be detained in hospital under Section 2 and Section 3 of the Mental Health Act [1].

** An 'approved mental health professional' (AMHP) is a social worker, mental health nurse, occupational therapist or psychologist who has received special training to help decide whether people need to be admitted to hospital. They are 'approved' by a local social services authority for five years at a time. Most AMHPs are social workers [1].

4.2 "Section?"

Candidate's Instructions:

You are the foundation year doctor working on the psychiatric inpatient unit doctor. Miles is a 70-year-old gentleman whose wife died one month ago. Soon after his mood became extremely low, he stopped eating and drinking, he became severely dehydrated and malnourished and was treated in hospital. When Paul was about to be discharged, he said that he plans to join his wife in heaven and attempted to hang himself in the ward bathroom. A Mental Health Act Assessment (MHAA) was held and Paul was placed on Section 2 of the MHA and transferred to a psychiatric hospital.

Paul feels better but wants to talk to you about the 'this Section business' and what it means for him. You have 8 minutes.

Examiner's Instructions

The foundation year doctor working on a psychiatric inpatient ward has been asked to see a 70-year-old gentleman called Miles. His wife died one month ago. Soon after his mood became extremely low, he stopped eating and drinking, he became severely dehydrated, and malnourished and was treated in hospital. When Miles was about to be discharged, he said that he plans to join his wife in heaven and attempted to hang himself in the ward bathroom. A Mental Health Act Assessment was held and Miles was placed on Section 2 of the MHA and transferred to a psychiatric hospital.

Miles feels better but wants to talk to the doctor about the 'this Section business' and what it means. The candidate has 8 minutes.

Pay careful attention to the language used by the candidate – avoid the use of jargon and be sensitive to patient's ignorance.

Candidate should be able to explain why a section is used, how long it can be used for, what reason there might be to use it, who is able to use it and what the patient can do to appeal the decision; for the most commonly used MHA sections.

Actor's instructions

Background:
You are a 70-year-old man called Miles. You were taken into hospital by your son and daughter. They have been very worried about you since your wife of 25 years died one month ago. After which you became increasingly depressed and suicidal, you stopped eating and drinking completely until you became very dehydrated and needed intravenous fluid rehydration. At that point you didn't feel you could go anymore. You attempted to hang himself in the ward bathroom in desperate attempt to end your suffering.

In the hospital your memory is hazy you remember being seen by the psychiatric team and being told you were under Section 2, but do not know what this means. You are very worried that you will be made to stay in hospital for a very long time.
You want to speak to the doctor to discuss these concerns.

Please ask the following questions regarding your Section 2;
- What is a Section?
- Why was it used?
- Who made that decision?
- How long does it last?
- What happens next?
- What can you do to challenge the decision?

Your mental state:
You have started to accept your wife's passing and your mood has lifted significantly. You have poor eye contact and stooped posture. Your speech is of normal volume, but slightly slower. You are eating and drinking adequately now.

Risk:

You no longer have suicidal thoughts and regret your attempt in hospital, you want to be alive to see your grandchildren grow up and know this is what your wife would want.

OSCE Station – 'Section?'

Task:	Achieved	Not Achieved
Introduces self		
Clarifies patient identity and gains consent		
Establishes rapport		
Asks open question to patient about concerns		
Explains what Section 2 is – Assessment of mental illness and need for hospital admission		
Explains why Section 2 is used – patient is deemed mentally ill and a risk to himself or others. Not previously been assessed in hospital before or not assessed for a long time.		
Explains who can decide to place someone under Section 2 – two fully registered doctors (one approved) working independently and one approved social worker		
Explains how long Section 2 lasts for – 28 days, cannot be renewed		
Explains what happens next – a decision will be made whether the patient should be placed on Section 3 – a treatment order lasting 6 months		
Explains that If patient disagrees with consultants' decision they are entitled to a tribunal meeting in front of a judge who will decide whether the patient should remain under section.		
Explains that patient can appeal against Section 2 in the first 14 days only.		
Your responsible clinician can discharge you from Section 2 at any time if he / she feels they are no longer a danger to themselves		
Reassures patient they will be assessed by a consultant regularly		
Explains that the patient can apply for an Independent Mental Health Advocate (IMHA) to help tell staff about their concerns		
Explains patient is entitled to free legal advice		
Asks about ideas, concerns and expectations		
Gives patient opportunity to ask questions		

Gives the patient some literature on section 2 and the appeal process		
Empathetic manner		
Non-judgmental approach		
Examiner's Global Mark	/5	
Actor / Helper's Global Mark	/5	
Total Station Mark	/30	

Learning Points

- The MHA was passed in 1983, and amended in 2007. It allows for the compulsory admission of those who are mentally ill. The most important parts for OSCE exams are Section 2, 3, 4, 5, and police Sections 135 and 136.

- Section 2 is an assessment order for 28 days, must be signed by 2 doctors and an Approved Mental Health Practitioner (AMHP). The 2 doctors are supposed to assess the patient within 5 hours of each other, and cannot be employed by the same organisation, i.e. have to be independent from each other.

- Patients detained under sections 2 and 3 have the right to appeal, and if they choose to appeal they will be presented to a tribunal panel, which consists of an independent psychiatrist, a judge and a lay-person.

4.3 "I am not having the op, doc"

Candidate's Instructions:

You are the foundation doctor on call and have been asked to see a patient called Joseph on the surgical ward. Joseph has a gangrenous foot and needs to have an emergency amputation to save his life.

The nurse on the ward tells you that Joseph appears to be low in mood, he is not eating his meals and rarely makes conversation. When she approached him to discuss the operation he told her he would not sign the consent form.

Please assess Joseph's capacity to consent to the amputation of his foot. You have 6 minutes after which you will be asked some questions.

Examiner's Instructions:

Joseph is a patient on the surgical ward who is refusing to sign a consent form for a potentially lifesaving emergency operation to remove his gangrenous foot.

The foundation year doctor on call has been asked to determine the patient's capacity to consent to the amputation of his foot. They have been told that nursing staff have noticed that Joseph appears to be low in mood, is not eating his meals and rarely makes conversation.

Pay particular attention to the candidate's interaction with the depressed and anxious patient.

At 6 minutes, ask the candidate to summarize the case, followed by their investigation and management plan.

Actor's Instructions:

Background

You are a 65-year-old called Joseph. English is your first language and you don't have any problems with your hearing or eye sight. Your wife died 2 years ago and you have one son who lives 1 hour away who "has his own family to worry about." You are concerned about becoming a burden. You are now retired, but previously worked as a mechanic and enjoyed staying active. These days you are housebound and can only walk for very short distances because of the pain in your foot.

You are a heavy smoker, don't drink much alcohol and you don't use drugs. You have no particular religious beliefs. You have not spoken to your son about the operation as you don't want to bother him, but you will agree for the doctor to call your son if she thinks it is useful. You have high cholesterol, hypertension, type 2 diabetes and have had two previous heart attacks. You have a long list of medication including insulin, but you cannot remember them all. You have no previous psychiatric history.

Behaviour

You are low in mood, downcast expression, forgetful at times and will ask for questions to be repeated, you are also finding it difficult to focus and will often reply "I don't know" or "I can't remember" in a hopeless fashion.

Capacity questions – when prompted

The problem: You understand that the circulation in your foot is very bad and the surgeon wants to remove it.

Advantages of amputation: You struggle to think of any advantages, but with reassurance and prompting you say it might stop the pain.

Disadvantages of amputation: When asked about disadvantages, you explain the surgeon went over some risks of not having the procedure but you can't remember what he said. Cannot recall the risks mentioned.

Towards the end you make a comment that you do not feel very talkative and are getting tired.

Mental state

You feel low and ambivalent about dying, sometimes wondering what's the point in carrying on. You have no active suicidal plans. You have not been eating and sleeping well. You used to like watching television but have stopped doing this as you struggled to follow the story and lose concentration. You deny delusions, auditory or visual hallucinations.

Capacity Assessment Station – "I'm not having the op doc"

Task:	Achieved	Not Achieved
Introduces self		
Clarifies who they are speaking to and obtains consent		
Establishes rapport		
Explores patient's understanding of the situation and why they do not want the operation		
Asks about advantages and disadvantages of the operation		
Asks patient if they can remember some of the risks of not undergoing the operation		
Helps patient to identify risks of not undergoing the operation (risk of losing more of the leg, risk of death, other sensible e.g. septicaemia, blood loss)		
Asks about depressive symptoms (low mood, anhedonia, fatigue, sleep, appetite, libido, concentration)		
Asks about self-harm or suicidal thoughts		
Asks about drug and alcohol use		
Asks about religious beliefs and impact		
Asks about family involvement and gains consent to discuss situation with next of kin		
Asks patient if they could have a second discussion on a different day		
Offers to leave further information about the procedure with the patient		
Assesses patient ideas, concerns and expectations		
Summarises consultation and decision making concisely (comments on understanding, retaining, weighing up and communicating)		
Correctly determines patient does not have capacity		
Provides management plan (ask for psychiatric opinion, discuss with surgeon - ?possibility if delaying surgery, suggest MMSE)		
Non coercive		
Non-judgmental approach		
Examiner's Global Mark	/5	
Actor / Helper's Global Mark	/5	
Total Station Mark	/30	

Learning Points

- The Mental Capacity Act (2005) consists of 5 key statutory principles

    1. Person is deemed to have capacity unless it is established that they do not.
    2. You must take PRACTICAL steps to help patients make a decision e.g. ask for interpreter, use visual aids.
    3. A person is allowed to make an unwise decision.
    4. If a decision is made for a person who lacks capacity, it must be made with their best interest in mind.
    5. The decision or act carried out must be completed in the least restrictive way possible.

- In order to assess this, you should ask the following questions. A failure in any one of these points makes a person non capacitous for that particular decision.

    Do they *understand* 'relevant information'?
    Are they able to *retain* this information?
    Are they able to *weigh up* that information as part of a decision making process?
    Can they *communicate* their decision back?

4.4 "I must have fallen..."

Candidate's Instructions:

You are the foundation year doctor working in the emergency department You are seeing a 35-year-old patient called Faye who has told you that she fell down the stairs. On examination, she has a black eye and a number of older looking bruises on her arms and chest. You don't feel these injuries fit with the story she gives you about falling down the stairs.

She tells you she has been feeling sick and dizzy recently and you decide to send her for CT scan of the head, however when the results come back as normal and you tell her she can go home she looks distressed and fearful.

Her presentation greatly concerns you. Please assess her further and explore her concerns. You have 7 minutes to do this, after which you will be asked some questions.

Examiner's Instructions:

The foundation year doctor has seen a 35-year-old patient in the emergency department called Faye. There are signs that this patient has been a victim of assault, possibly domestic violence (DV). The foundation year doctor should have picked up on these signs and screen for DV. The doctor should attempt build a rapport with the patient in a non-judgmental and caring manner and ask about the different types of abuse tactfully. The doctor should not assume that the patient will want to leave their partner or make demands of this nature to the patient.

The doctor should assess immediate and long term risk to patient and other family members. The doctor should be supportive and offer sensible advice e.g. call the police. The doctor could suggest admitting the patient overnight if there are felt to be immediate risks.

At 7 minutes, please stop the candidate and discuss their management plan. The doctor should discuss with senior colleagues and seek advice about who else they need to contact, such as DV liaison nurse.

Actor's Instructions:

Background

You are a 35-year-old called Faye. You are not married but your boyfriend is very abusive and has repeatedly punched you in the face and head, you have started to feel dizzy and sick and you are worried he might have done permanent damage. Reluctantly he allows you to go and get checked out at the emergency department and you secretly hope you are admitted overnight for a break. You do want to talk to somebody about getting help but you are worried your partner might find out.

History of symptoms

You have one child with your boyfriend who is 2 years old. Since her birth the abuse has got progressively worse with weekly assaults. He usually kicks, punches or slaps you. He has never sexually abused you. Your family is supportive and they are worried about you. They do not get on with your partner and he does not like you to see them. You have stopped going out to see family members or friends to avoid confrontation. Your family are not aware of the physical abuse and you feel too ashamed to tell them.

You do not have any medical problems, take regular medications or have allergies. You have never had any contact with the mental health services. You work as a project manager and have supportive work colleagues.

Risk

Your partner recently lost his job and is drinking alcohol more frequently he is more aggressive when drunk and this is when you feel most at risk, he gets drunk 2-3 times per week. You are not aware of him owning any weapons. You do not self harm but have had fleeting suicidal thoughts in the past, but know you would never act on these thoughts in order to take care of your daughter. You do not drink or take drugs. You are sure that your partner has never in the past been abusive towards your daughter but you are worried about what she might have seen or heard and what impact this is having. Currently, your daughter is safe with your mother.

If you go home, there is a chance your partner will be drunk you were hoping to stay the night and return home in the morning. You would be open to speaking with a DV nurse on the ward.

Capacity Assessment Station – "I must have fallen…"

Task:	Achieved	Not Achieved
Introduces self		
Clarifies who they are speaking to and gains consent		
Establishes rapport		
Assures patient of confidentiality / privacy		
Uses open ended questions "how are things at home?" (nature, onset, triggers, timing, exacerbating factors)		
Raises concern in non-judgmental manner "I'm concerned about your safety"		
Makes empathetic and supportive remarks "it's not your fault"		
Screens for different types of abuse; physical / sexual / emotional / neglect		
Establishes frequency of abuse		
Determines social situation (home, family, relationships, employment) and support network.		
Ask about partners drug / alcohol abuse in relation to risk		
Determine patient's drug or alcohol use "How are you coping?"		
Asks if there are any weapons in the house		
Asks about self-harm and suicidality		
Asks about mood and depressive symptoms (low mood, anhedonia, fatigue, appetite, concentration)		
Explores risk to others; specifically the daughter		
Establishes that daughter is currently safe with her grandmother		
Give sensible advice – call the police, speak with a family member, admit overnight, refer to local domestic abuse service		
Explains you will have to inform social services about the children		
Discusses case with a senior medic		

Examiner's Global Mark	/5	
Actor / Helper's Global Mark	/5	
Total Station Mark	/30	

Learning Points

- Domestic violence (DV) is more common than we think, 1 in 4 women and 1 in 6 men will be affected during their lifetime. Suffers of DV are more likely to suffer with chronic illness, mental health problems, and addiction. It is most important to screen for these.

- If a patient reports abuse to a child or vulnerable adult who lacks capacity, then you are obligated to report this to social services even if the patinet is unhappy about this.

- It is important to give the patient practical advice about how to seek help .In the UK there is a free phone 24 hour national domestic violence helpline 0808 2000 247. You do not have to speak English to use this service.

4.5 "He deserved it"

Candidate's Instructions:

You are a foundation year doctor working for a Psychiatry Liaison Team in a District General Hospital. You have been asked to assess a 35-year-old man called Jamie on the surgical ward who has assaulted another patient because "the voices told me to." They would like a psychiatry opinion.

Please take a history from the patient of the index offence, focusing on forensic history, with a view to establishing a likely diagnosis. You have 6 minutes to take the history, after which you will be asked some questions.

Examiner's Instructions:

The candidate is a foundation year doctor working with a Liaison Psychiatry team in a District General Hospital. They have been asked to take a history from a patient called Jamie on the surgical ward, who has assaulted another patient because "the voices told me to."

Please stop the candidate at 6 minutes in order to ask some further questions.

1. **QUESTION: What do you think is the most likely diagnosis?**
   History and presentation all suggest to antisocial personality disorder: Behaviour as an adolescent leading to detention in a young offender's institution; multiple convictions for assault; lack of interpersonal relationships; lack of remorse; inability to accept responsibility for his problems or antisocial behaviour.

2. **QUESTION: Is there anything we should rule out?**
   Need to rule out a psychotic element, as patient says he is hearing voices (however no features of "true" psychosis; voices are experienced as internal and not real). Consider acute delirium as patient recently underwent an appendectomy. If he has left the ward for any period, it is worth considering acute alcohol or drug intoxication as a contributing factor given his history.

3. **QUESTION: What advice would you give to the ward about managing this man's behaviour?**
   Essentially, unless there is another reason to doubt this man's capacity (e.g. if he were acutely delirious) any antisocial behaviour should be referred to the police. The patient is medically ready to be discharged therefore could be taken into police custody if necessary.

Actor's Instructions:

Background:
You are a 35-year-old man called Jamie on an acute surgical ward, recovering from acute appendicitis. You have been aggressive towards another patient, and the candidate has been asked to take a history from you.

Incident:
You got into a fight with another patient on the ward who was shouting for the nurses and irritating you. You feel he started it and that your response was justified, and you do not feel guilty. You heard a male voice saying "go on, just do it, hit him, you know you want to, that'll shut him up!" You know this voice came from inside your head and you knew it was not real. In a flush of anger, you punched him.

Your history of symptoms:
You have no long-term medical conditions and do not take any regular medication. You have previously been assessed by the children's mental health team at the age of 15. You were discharged – you don't know if you were diagnosed with anything. You don't think you have a mental illness. If asked, you often hear voices telling you to do things – you experience these as in your head, and you know they are not real. You have never been on antipsychotic medications or antidepressants.

You were brought up by your grandparents; you never knew your father (he and you mother separated before you were born), and your mother had problems with drug use. You attended mainstream schools but never did well – you got into trouble for truancy, and at the age of 15 you stopped attending altogether.
You have worked on and off, in various manual labour posts. You have never had a relationship. You currently live alone in a bed-sit. You manage financially with help from your grandparents, who you see occasionally.

You have been in prison many times – maybe 6 or 7, including six months at a young offender's institute. The crimes have all been assault, Actual Bodily Harm (ABH) or theft. You feel you have not been justly treated. No known mental illness in your family history other than your mother's substance misuse. You drink alcohol in a "binge pattern" (sometimes up to 10 pints in one sitting) but not every day. You do not use other drugs.

Your behaviour:
Your manner is defensive and sometimes hostile, although you co-operate. Your arms are crossed in a defensive manner. You do not accept responsibility for any of your behaviour – rather, you feel the other party is responsible. You have never liked other people or formed any close friendships; if asked about your relationship with your grandparents, be dismissive. You have a poor opinion of the NHS in general. You do not feel depressed.

Antisocial PD – "He deserved it"

Task:	Achieved	Not Achieved
Introduces self		
Clarifies who they are speaking to and gains consent		
Establishes rapport		
Establishes patient's version of altercation with other patients (nature, onset, triggers, timing, exacerbating factors)		
Enquires about nature of voices		
Asks about other psychotic symptoms (hallucinations, illusions)		
Establishes the patient's reaction to it – feels justified, no guilt or remorse		
Establishes past psychiatric history including contact with CAMHS.		
Establishes past medical history (nil, other than this current admission for appendicitis).		
Social History: Establishes current housing and work		
Social History: Establishes lack of relationships		
Enquires about forensic history		
Substance Use: Establishes drinking pattern and asks about other substances.		
Personal History: Enquires about childhood and early life		
Establishes past medical history (nil, other than this current admission for appendicitis).		
Risk assessment (to self, to others, from others)		
QUESTION 1: Most likely diagnosis is antisocial personality disorder		
QUESTION 2: Need to rule out intoxication, psychosis, delirium		
QUESTION 3: Medication not indicated; police should be involved		
Non-judgmental approach		

Examiner's Global Mark	/5	
Actor / Helper's Global Mark	/5	
Total Station Mark	/30	

Learning Points

- A personality disorder is defined as: "Enduring maladaptive patterns of behaviour, cognition, and inner experience... deviating markedly from those accepted by the individual's culture". Research suggests that personality disorders fall into three groups. This has colloquially been described for revision purposes as "mad, bad and sad"

- Cluster A: 'Odd or eccentric' e.g. paranoid, schizoid – MAD
- Cluster B: 'dramatic, emotional or erratic' e.g. antisocial, emotionally unstable, narcissistic – BAD
- Cluster C: 'anxious and fearful' e.g. obsessive-compulsive, avoidant – SAD

- Antisocial personality disorder is characterized by impulsive, deviant behavior, disrespect for societal norms, lack of remorse and a disregard for the rights and welfare of other people.

- Patients with an antisocial personality disorder often come the way of general adult psychiatry services as well as forensic services. It is very common to be asked to assess such patients regarding their capacity or whether they are suffering from an acute mental illness. Their risk to others must be well documented, and discussed with forensic services as necessary. It is important to establish comorbities such as psychosis or substance misuse in order to correctly recommend treatment.

4.6 "Lady in red"

Candidate's Instructions:

You are a foundation year doctor on call covering a psychiatric inpatient hospital. You have been called to see a 42-year-old man called Derek in the Section 136 Suite in the emergency department. He was found shouting, threatening and fighting with two members of public whilst in possession of a knife. The police felt he was mentally unwell and brought him to ED handcuffed.

Please take a history from the patient of the index offence, with a view to establishing a likely diagnosis and risk assessment.

You have 6 minutes to take the history after which the examiner will ask you some questions.

Examiner's Instructions:

The candidate is an F2 on call covering a psychiatric inpatient hospital. They have been called to the Section 136 Suite in the emergency department see a 42-year-old man called Derek, who was brought in by the police. The man was shouting at his wife and another member of public in the street. He was aggressive, fighting, waving a knife, and was felt to be mentally unwell.

The candidate's task is to take a focused history with a view to establishing a diagnosis, including a brief risk assessment.

Please stop them after 7 minutes to ask the following questions:

1. What do you think is the most likely diagnosis? (Delusional Disorder/ Othello Syndrome)
2. What is your risk assessment? (Must mention significant risk to others, specifically his wife – also note young children at home)
3. What would your immediate management plan be? (Physical examination, bloods, ECG, urine drug screen, search patient for weapons)

Actor's Instructions:

Background:
You are a 42-year-old man called Derek who has been brought into the emergency department by the police. You were shouting in the street and waving a knife at your wife (the doctor does not know she is your wife initially) and another member of public.

Your current beliefs:
You are suffering from delusions of jealousy: You "know" your wife is having an affair. You interpret everything thing your wife says and does (e.g. going out with friends) as infidelity. You think this has been going on for about 6 months – you don't know who the other party is but you suspect it is someone from work. Your reasons for this belief are vague; e.g you think her manner towards you has changed. You have been going through your wife's belongings, reading her texts and following her to work in an attempt to get proof, all of which you are open about. Once you noticed she had purchased a new red dress, which must have meant she was unfaithful. Another time, you saw an unusual purchase on her credit card, which again, confirms her affair. You have confronted her about it more than once and she has vehemently denied it, but you know she is lying. You are arguing a lot. She has told you she is worried about you and that you should see a doctor. Recently, you have been carrying around a knife in case you track down the man who your wife is having an affair with.

Index offence:
Your wife told you she would be staying late at work. You waited outside her office to follow her home. You took a knife with you with the intent of threatening her and her boyfriend. She saw you following her and you lost control. Another member of the public got involved who and you threw punches at eachother. He is now pressing charges. You think you would have hurt her in anger. You have no thoughts or plans to harm yourself.

Your situation:
You have no psychiatric history. You have high cholesterol and are on medication for this. You have never been in trouble with the police and you have never behaved violently or aggressively before. You live with your wife of ten years, and your two children aged 4 and 8. You have no thoughts of anger or aggression towards your children. You work full-time as a chef, so you are usually busy in the evenings, but your preoccupation with your wife's infidelity has distracted you from your work. You have never used drugs but recently you have been drinking more alcohol than usual: 3-4 pints of lager most nights after work.

Your behaviour:
Your manner should be agitated, but you can hold a coherent conversation and have no other unusual beliefs, delusions or hallucinations. Your delusions are that they are completely fixed with no room for rational doubt, so everything you say should be said with certainty: "I know" rather than "I think". You believe all your actions have been entirely justified.

Morbid Jealousy

Task:	Achieved	Not Achieved
Introduces self		
Confirms patient identity and gains consent		
Establishes rapport		
Asks about the details of altercation in the street, and establishes the other party was his wife		
Establishes belief that his wife has been having an affair for past 6 months.		
Establishes that he lacks any proof but remains convinced		
Establishes patient's recent "stalking" behaviour: following his wife to work, going through her belongings, checking her phone and personal bills		
Enquires about other symptoms e.g other specific delusions, paranoia, hallucinations, illusions		
Enquires about Past Psychiatric History		
Asks about family history, including specifically about mental health and suicide		
Enquires about Past Medical History, medications, allergies and compliance		
Asks about social history (alcohol, smoking, drugs, employment, children)		
Enquires about Alcohol and Drugs		
Enquires about Forensic History		
Enquires about risk to self (thoughts of self-harm/ suicide, a history of self-harm)		
Establishes risk to others (has never been physically violent before, feelings of anger/ violence towards his wife currently, to children)		
Enquires about risk from others		
Question 1: Likely diagnosis? – Allow "Delusional Disorder", "Delusional Jealousy", "Morbid Jealousy"		
Question 2: One mark for recognition of significant risk to wife, could mention children at home/ increased alcohol intake.		

Question 3: Two marks for sensible plan – e.g admit patient, risk too high for home treatment. Could also include ruling out an organic cause, collateral history		
Examiner's Global Mark	/5	
Actor / Helper's Global Mark	/5	
Total Station Mark	/30	

Learning Points

- Morbid Jealousy, also known as "Othello Syndrome", is a type of Delusional Disorder; the patient presents with prominent delusions but WITHOUT accompanying hallucinations, thought disorder or significant mood disturbance.

- The key feature of Morbid Jealousy is a delusional belief in the partner's infidelity; this will be persistent over time and will be held with fixed intensity despite lack of evidence.

- Common behaviour includes:
  Checking on the partner: reading their messages, following them, going through their belongings
  Constantly questioning the partner's behaviour.
  Limiting the partner's freedom or isolating them from friends or family.

- Morbid Jealousy is associated with high risk of violence towards the partner, particularly when the patient is male. Other risks include violence towards the supposed third party, and children being witness to violence or abuse. As such, an automatic safeguarding alert would be completed.

Substance Misuse & Learning Disability (LD)

5.1 "Work hard, play hard"

Candidate's Instructions:

You are a foundation year doctor based in a GP surgery. A 26-year-old accountant called Wayne has attended the practice due to work related stress. He has been registered at the practice for the last 3 years but not been in to see anyone before.

Please take a history from Wayne. You have 7 minutes to do so after which you will be asked to summarise your findings to the GP.

Examiner's Instructions:

A 26 year old accountant called Wayne has attended the GP surgery due to work related stress. They have been registered at the practice for the last 3 years but been in to see anyone before.

The foundation year doctor based at the practice has been asked to take a history from this patient, with a view to summarize the findings back to the GP. The patient will let the doctor know that they have to go back to work urgently and may not be able to stay long

At 6 minutes, the patient insists they have to leave but will make another appointment towards the end of the week to discuss. Ask the candidate, for a summary and a management plan they would want to discuss with the patient when they reattend.

Actor's Instructions:

Background:
You are a 26-year-old accountant called Wayne. Your work has suggested you make an appointment to see your GP as you have had several days off "ill" in the last 3 months. Work are not aware of this, but you have had to take days off as you have been too hungover to go in. You are open about this. One of these sick days was an important presentation to a client.

>Your behaviour:
You are nervous and try to put on a jokey bravado - "I'm not really ill", "work just want me to come", "everyone in the city drinks a bit too much". You are keen for reassurance. You are cooperative generally, but you do not feel you need to seek any help yourself. You need to meet a client and are already late, so you tell the doctor at the beginning you need to go in about five minutes but you will make another appointment later in the week if they think you need to.

Your history of symptoms:
You started drinking aged 16 with friends. You like wine and beer but recently switched to spirits. You are on a prestigious graduate programme with a top London accountancy firm. Your work colleagues have a "work hard party hard" motto. You all go out most evenings after work. You always end up drunk. You enjoy the atmosphere, and feel like it is an extended "university" experience. You use the weekends to "recover."

In the last 6 months, you have noticed that your hands shake and you feel really sick in the mornings. Alcohol does not have the same effect as it used to and you have to drink more to get "drunk". You no longer like to have "drink free days" and on the weekends you would usually make sure some of your socialising is done in a bar. You are drinking about 4-5 pints of beer, 2-3 glasses of wine and few shots of whisky each day. Your partner gets annoyed with you and complained they have found you passed out in the morning on the stairs instead of in bed. They feel you are quick to get angry. You have never been violent or harmed others when drunk. You do not feel low, or suicidal.

You don't take any illicit drugs. You used to be avid rock climber but rarely go out now. You are not low but get irritated easily. You don't sleep much because of your partying. You eat less now that you are drinking so much alcohol. You have had no thoughts of hurting yourself or anyone else. You have no known medical problems and do not take any medications. No relevant family history.

You get annoyed if people mention your drinking. Eventually you admit there may be a problem with your drinking but you don't know what to do about it.

Alcohol STATION OSCE – "work hard, play hard"

Task:	Achieved	Not Achieved
Introduces self		
Confirms patient identity and obtains consent		
Establishes rapport		
Elicits history of drinking behaviour and pattern concisely (what, when, why, how much)		
CAGE questionnaire (do you think you need to cut down, has anyone ever got angry at you, do you feel guilty, have you ever had an eye opener)		
Establishes Dependence (psychological & physical) – including control, cravings, salience in life, tolerance, withdrawal symptoms, understanding of harm		
Asks about risky behaviours – driving, children, violence when drunk, been in risky situations, alcohol related crime		
Asks about other illicit drug use		
Abstinence: have you tried to stop? Previous attempts? Desire to stop?		
Screen for depression (low mood, anhedonia, fatigue)		
Screen for anxiety symptoms		
Asks about past psychiatric history		
Asks about medication history, allergies		
Asks about past medical history		
Asks about social history and impact on this (smoking, drugs, relationships, hobbies, employment)		
Asks about family history, including specifically about mental health and suicide		
Performs a risk assessment in a sensitive manner (to self, to others)		
Reassures patient when they try to leave, explains importance of assessment, and is positive		
Summarises consultation concisely		

Explains basic steps for management (reassurance, support, Alcohol services, AA, need for detox (community Vs residential)]		
Examiner's Global Mark	/5	
Actor / Helper's Global Mark	/5	
Total Station Mark	/30	

Learning Points:

- Alcohol dependence has wide reaching consequences to all aspects of people's lives. It is important to highlight and explore the impact this is having in all areas. People with alcohol dependence often have co-morbid psychiatric conditions, such as depression and anxiety. It is important to ask screening questions about this.

- The CAGE questionnaire is a useful screening test for alcoholism.
- To put things in perspective, a score of greater than or equal to 2 has a specificity of 77% and a sensitivity of 91% for the identification of alcoholism [1]. The ICD-10 diagnostic criteria for alcohol dependence is a useful reference when exploring alcohol traits with patients. The acronym WITCCH can be used to help you remember the components:

- Ask about **Withdrawal symptoms**
- Ask about the **Importance** of alcohol to their life (or salience), do they neglect pleasures or interests
- Ask about whether they need to drink more to get the same effect, or **Tolerance**
- Ask about **Cravings**
- Ask about whether they feel in **Control** of their drinking
- Ask about their understanding of **Harmful consequences**

- Demonstrating non-judgement and empathy is key in trying to explore some one's alcohol use. Offer to bring the patient back regularly (weekly perhaps) to support them in exploring and tackling their issue.

5.2 "Acutely under the influence"

Candidate's Instructions:

You are the foundation year doctor in the emergency department. A 20-year-old girl called Jade has been brought in by ambulance with injuries after having fallen from a first floor balcony. She is agitated, confused, angry and is holding her arm at a strange angle. The notes from the ambulance record say that the paramedics suspect the patient has been taking drugs. Jade has also lashed out and assaulted one of the paramedics.

Your registrar has asked you to take a history from this patient before discussing with them. You have 7 minutes to do so.

Examiner's Instructions

A 20-year-old female called Jade has been brought into the emergency department by ambulance with injuries after having fallen from a first floor balcony. She is agitated, confused and angry and holding their arm at a strange angle. She is acutely intoxicated after taking spice, GBL and crystal meth. She also lashed out and assaulted one of the paramedics on her way to A&E in the ambulance. The foundation year doctor in the emergency department who has been asked to assess the patient and report back to their registrar.

End the station at 7 minutes and ask the candidate to summarise, and ask them how they may proceed to try and assess the patient.

Actor's Instructions

Background:
You are a 20-year-old student called Jade. You have been out partying this whole weekend at a festival with friends. You have been taking a number of party drugs including smoking spice, GBL tablets & injecting crystal meth. You were at a friend's house when you suddenly thought you saw a snake and ran out to the balcony and jumped off to escape the snake. You remember hitting your head and your arm.

You have a headache and have vomited once. Your arm is unbearably painful and you cannot straighten it. You hold it hugged into your chest. Your friends called an ambulance but you don't really remember much except hitting your head against the floor and that your arm really hurts and you cannot move it. You often take party drugs at the weekend with friends but this is the first time you have taken such a large quantity over a short space of time. You have never hallucinated before. You usually just feel really "alive" and exhilarated.

When you are not taking drugs you feel fine. Today you are scared, paranoid, jumpy, keep thinking you see a snake and are very angry. Your thoughts are disordered.

Your behaviour:
Throughout the consultation: "get away from me. I'll F*****G punch you if you come near me!" "I just want to go home", "What the F*** do you know? who are you? " "Can't you see it? It's just there, the snake". You are extremely agitated. You have a headache. The lights in A&E are too bright. You are angry and shout a lot. You keep seeing colours in the room. You think you see a snake near where the doctor is standing and this snake has followed you from your friend's house. You want to go home. You are in pain but you think all you need is to "sleep off" the bad trip you are having. You don't want anyone to touch you. You are

abusive to the doctor and swear a lot. You also scream intermittently that the pain in your arm is unbearable. You are quite confused and will randomly say odd words out of context (e.g. snake, wired, shakes). You refuse all medical help or attempts at examination or intervention. You refuse to sit down, pacing around the room. You try and leave the room several times but respond to the doctor's attempts to get you to stay. You say personally derogatory things to the doctor to try get them to react to you. **You attempt to pick up the chair and threaten to throw it at the doctor at one point.** If the doctor approaches you in a calm and soothing manner, you may calm down temporarily.

The doctor may try and get you to sit down or ask to examine you. You react violently to this suggestion. If they say they will have to end the consultation or call security you temporarily calm down.

OCD STATION OSCE – "acutely under the influence

Task:	Achieved	Not Achieved
Introduces self		
Confirms patient identity and gains consent		
Establishes rapport		
Calm in manner, trying to de-escalate situation		
Establishes sequence of events		
Establish what substances they have taken, route of administration, any drugs or alcohol with them, and how long ago		
Asks if equipment is shared		
Asks how drugs are obtained, and paid for		
Establish what injuries they may have now		
Asks about psychotic symptoms (hallucinations, delusions, thought insertion / withdrawal / broadcast)		
Asks about history of drug and alcohol use		
Asks about impact of patients drug use on: physical health, mental health, social / family life, financial and legal matters		
Asks about past medical history		
Asks about past psychiatric history, previous overdoses etc		
Asks about medication, allergies and compliance.		
Asks about social history including social support network (family / friends)		
Performs a risk assessment - safety to self, others, staff. Call for help if needed (security guard, terminating consultation, seeking help from seniors or others)		
Reassures patient when they try to leave, explains importance of assessment and concerns they have		

Summarises consultation concisely		
Explains basic steps for next steps of management including mentioning rapid tranquillisation		
Examiner's Global Mark	/5	
Actor / Helper's Global Mark	/5	
Total Station Mark	/30	

Learning Points

- It is important to remain calm in a heightened situation with a patient. Remember your non-verbal communication skills such as body language, eye contact, personal space. Never put yourself at risk; if you feel you are, indicate you will need to ask security or others to come help you for the safety of yourself and the patient. Your safety comes first.

- People who are acutely intoxicated may lack capacity temporarily - in this case, this patient may be significantly injured but unable to understand this. They may need to be medically calmed down using rapid tranquilisation to allow a better assessment in the patient's best interests. This would always be a team decision and you should involve your seniors.

- After discussing with your seniors, check your local prescribing guidelines for rapid tranquillisation, a common first line is lorazepam. You should always consider oral before intramuscular as this is least restrictive.

5.3 "Desiring diazepam"

Candidate's Instructions:

You're a foundation year doctor in a GP surgery. A 40-year-old woman called Nikki attends the practice for a review. The notes say that she has a history of heroin dependence, and alcohol misuse. She has presented regularly in the last year seeking benzodiazepines for anxiety. There is a clear note from one of the GPs who saw him last week, stating that they were concerned that this patient was developing dependence and this should be explored at the next review.

Please take a history from this patient and explore his concerns. You have 7 minutes to do this, after which you will be asked for your management plan.

Examiner's Instructions:

A 40-year-old-female called Nikki attends the GP surgery for a review. The notes say that she has a history of heroin dependence and alcohol misuse. She has presented regularly in the last year seeking benzodiazepines for anxiety. There is a clear note from one of the GPs who saw her last week, stating that there was concern this patient was developing a dependence and this should be explored at the next review.

The candidate is a foundation year doctor at the GP surgery who is booked to see this patient. They have 7 minutes after which please ask them for their management plan.

They should assess the patient's current problems, explore their concerns and make a management plan with the patient (this could include another appointment to discuss further, talking about treating underlying depression or anxiety, psychological work, referral to drug service or working to reduce diazepam use at the surgery).

Actor's instructions

Background:
You are a 40-year-old called Nikki. You have a long history of heroin and alcohol misuse. You have been in and out of drug services for many years but 5 years ago you managed to achieve abstinence after a prolonged period of detoxification and rehabilitation. However, since coming out you have been feeling very anxious all the time and started taking diazepam, which has been helpful.

Your behaviour:
You are anxious and fidgety in your presentation. You are proud that you have managed to stop using drugs and turned your life around and are reluctant to see your current use as a problem or be labelled as a "druggie". You get irritated and angry if the doctor suggests that you may have a "problem". If the doctor is calm, non-judgemental and empathetic to your issues, you calm down and are amenable to speaking about a plan of action.

Your history of symptoms:
You have a long history of drug use that started in your teens. Your parents were both drug users. You have been with drug services on and off for many years. You used to drink up to 1 litre of whisky a day and inject £100 of heroin daily. You begged for money and stole to fund your drug habit. You have been arrested for shop lifting and served a 2-month prison sentence for this. From prison you entered a detoxification and rehabilitation programme and have managed to remain abstinent for five years. You attend Narcotic Anonymous (NA) twice per week.

You live alone and are single. You were in a relationship until last year but this broke down after your partner cheated on you. You have been lonely since then and your confidence has been destroyed. After the breakdown of this relationship, you noticed you felt low and anxious when you were in crowds. You can't sleep at night because you ruminate on thoughts that you are useless.

You are not suicidal. You found it difficult to leave the house to attend your NA meetings and to do your volunteer work at the homeless shelter. You saw a GP about a year ago who gave a short supply of diazepam 5mg three per day to help with anxiety and sleep. This was really helpful. Since then you have increased to 30mg a day. You admit that you are worried about becoming dependent but you don't know what to do. Your greatest fear is that you will start to turn to a dealer to get diazepam and that could spiral into your previous lifestyle. You tried to stop once for a day but felt too sick.

Questions and actions:
Throughout the consultation: "it'll be the end if I'm dependent on drugs again", "I don't have a problem, I just need to get through the day", "I can't cope if you stop my diazepam doctor!"

OSCE – Use of Harmful Substances

Task:	Achieved	Not Achieved
Introduces self		
Confirms patient identity and gains consent		
Establishes rapport		
Elicits presenting complaint		
Explores diazepam use – what, when, how, why, quantity		
Establishes Dependence (psychological & physical) – cravings, sweating, anxiety		
Explores related risks: route of use, using illicitly, how are they funding it, driving whilst on it, looking after children or working with vulnerable people whilst under the influence		
Explores other illicit drug or alcohol use		
Explores impact on social circumstances (relationships, physical health, sleep, interests, work)		
Explores abstinence: have you tried to stop? Previous attempts? Desire to stop? History of fits on stopping?		
Asks about co-morbid low mood (low mood, anhedonia, fatigue)		
Asks about co-morbid anxiety symptoms		
Asks about past medical history		
Asks about past psychiatric history		
Asks about medication history, allergies and compliance		
Performs a risk assessment in a sensitive manner		
Explains concerns to patient in non-judgmental way and in clear simple terms		
Explores patient's concerns and fears appropriately		
Summarises consultation & actions from here on		
Creates an appropriate joint management plan to support patient. Talks about referral to drug service +/- plan to reduce diazepam sensibly in GP surgery. Discusses other treatments for underlying anxiety & depression		
Examiner's Global Mark	/5	

Actor / Helper's Global Mark	/5	
Total Station Mark	/30	

Learning Points:

- Approaching the patient in a non-judgmental and empathetic manner is key to establishing the concerns and issues here and getting the patient alongside.

- People often use illicit substances to treat co-morbid or underlying psychiatric symptoms; it is vital to screen for these and think about treatment of this alongside treatment of drug dependence.

- Creating a joint plan that seems manageable and supportive for the patient is key – get them to think about suggest things that they have found helpful in the past or may find helpful now.

5.4 "Experimenting"

Candidate's Instructions:

You're the foundation year doctor at the GP surgery. A 19-year-old female called Stacey attends the practice as they have recently started university in the area. She has booked in to ask for the morning after pill after she had a night out under the influence of club drugs. This is her first appointment at the practice.

Please take a history from Stacey, focusing on her illicit drug use history. You have 7 minutes to do so after which you will be asked to discuss your concerns with Stacey and suggest a management plan.

Examiner's Instructions:

A 19 year old patient called Stacey attends the GP surgery. She is new to the surgery as she has recently started university in the area. She has booked in to ask for the morning after pill. She is using GBL and mephedrone since starting university, whilst at parties. Yesterday she had sex with someone unknown whilst high and are now worried they may be pregnant and / or "caught something".

The candidate is a foundation year doctor at the GP surgery who is booked to see Stacey. They should assess the patient's current problems, explore their concerns and make a joint management plan with the patient (this could include another appointment to discuss further, psycho-education around using club drugs, harm reduction advice and discussion, advice about seeking further help).

The candidate has 7 minutes to take the history, after which they should be asked for their management plan.

Actor's Instructions:

Background:
You are a 19-year-old student called Stacey studying for a Law degree. Yesterday you had unprotected sex with a stranger whilst high at a party, after taking mephedrone and GBL. You are worried about getting pregnant and "catching something". You came to the GP surgery to ask for the morning after pill. When asked about what happened, you are open about using club drugs.

History of symptoms:
You started university a few months ago. You have been having an amazing time, exploring who are you, making new friends and partying. You have experimented with club drugs and have really liked the experience. You are usually shy, so the drugs make you "get into the swing of things". You cannot party without them now.

Your friends introduced you to clubs drugs a few months ago. You have tried LSD, ketamine, cocaine, GBL, mephedrone and crystal meth. You have tried cannabis in the past too but this made you "paranoid" so you stopped. You have never tried heroin. You have taken these substances orally and smoked but never injected anything. You have shared crack pipes before with people at parties. You like the "high" and the sense of "being one with everything" when you take these drugs. You sometimes need a "pick me up" in the middle of the week to "get you through" to the weekend. You have had unprotected sex previously whilst high and have woken up in random people's bed with no recollection of what happened the night before. This had not worried you before as; "it's part of the Uni experience, right?"

You like your course and have wanted to be lawyer for as long as you can remember. Your parents are also lawyers. You have a group of close friends at Uni. Recently you have been falling behind on assignments. You failed one essay last month which is unusual for you. You got irritated when a friend said she thought you were taking too many drugs. You are open to the idea you may need help of some sort and accepting of coming back to see GP and maybe seeing a club drug service. You do not have any mental health or medical problems, take any regular medications, or have allergies.

Your behaviour:
You are embarrassed but also anxious. If the doctor is sensitive and encouraging, you easily unburden your worries and troubles. If you feel they are judgmental, you are dismissive of their advice and just want the "morning after pill".

You don't feel low. You have had enjoyable hallucinations on the drugs before. You sometimes feel tired mid-week but if you use drugs again it helps you get through until the weekend. You have no problems with your sleep. You have had no thoughts about hurting yourself. You get more easily irritated recently.

Questions and actions:
Throughout the consultation: "everyone does it right?", "Uni is there for experimentation?"

OSCE – Use of Harmful Substances

Task:	Achieved	Not Achieved
Introduces self		
Confirms patient identity and gains consent		
Establishes rapport		
Elicits presenting complaint: wants morning after pill after having unprotected sex under the influence of club drugs		
Establishes what drugs are they using		
Establishes route of intake, amount & how long they have been using		
Explores other illicit drug or alcohol use		
Explores impact on social circumstances (relationships, physical health, sleep, interests and work, finances)		
Explores abstinence: have you tried to stop? Previous attempts? Desire to stop?		
Establishes dependence (psychological & physical) – cravings, sweating, anxiety		
Asks about co-morbid low mood (low mood, anhedonia, fatigue)		
Asks about co-morbid anxiety symptoms		
Asks about past medical history		
Asks about past psychiatric history		
Asks about medication history and allergies		
Performs a risk assessment: how are they funding the habit, any overdoses, sharing any equipment, unprotected sex, BBV screening, thoughts to harm self or others		
Counsels patient appropriately on concerns, possible consequences of continued drug use.		
Mentions harm minimisation behaviours (contraception including condoms, Gum clinic screening, BBV immunisations)		
Explores patient's concerns and fears appropriately and in a non-judgmental manner		

Creates an appropriate joint management plan to support patient. Further appointments & discusses possible referral to club drugs clinic		
Examiner's Global Mark	/5	
Actor / Helper's Global Mark	/5	
Total Station Mark	/30	

Learning Points:

- Thinking with the patient about the good and bad things about using drugs is a good way to explore the issue with a patient who maybe ambivalent about their use.

- It is important to think laterally about your risk assessment with these patients and a key part of your management is harm reduction techniques (i.e. using disposable needles, not sharing equipment, having BBV immunisations, contraception etc.) followed by bringing them back for reassessment.

- When taking a drug history, you may have to specifically ask about different types of drugs (i.e. running through a list) as some people will not consider novel psychoactive substances (NPS – formally known as "legal highs", of which there are over 100), club drugs, cannabis, or prescription medication as "real drugs".Below is a crib sheet of common classifications of drugs, examples, and route of administration.

Classification	Common Drugs	Route
Opioids (depressants)	Heroin, opium, codeine	Smoked, snorted, swallowed, IV
Stimulants	Cocaine / crack	Snorted, smoked, IV
	Amphetamine	Swallowed, smoked, snorted, IV
	Meta-amphetamines	Swallowed, smoked, snorted, IV
Hallucinogenic	LSD	Swallowed/ absorbed

	Psilocybin (magic mushrooms)	swallowed
Club drugs	MDMA	IV swallowed, snorted
	GHB / GBL	IV swallowed
	Flunitrazepam (Rohypnol)	IV swallowed, snorted
Cannaboids	Cannabis/ Marijuana/ hash	Smoked, swallowed
Novel Psychoactive Substances (NPS – formally known as "legal highs")	Innumerable examples: spice, black mamba, mephedrone, kryptonite, chronic etc.	Swallowed, snorted, smoked, IV

5.5 "Change in behaviour"

Candidate's Instructions:

You are a foundation year doctor based in a GP surgery. A parent has made an appointment with the GP to discuss their 24-year-old son, Jacob, who has a mild-to moderate learning disability (LD). Jacob has been known and followed up by the LD team since childhood. Recently his parents, who are his carers, have noticed some challenging behaviour. He is not present at this appointment as he is scared of doctors.

Please explore, assess and address the parent's concerns. You have 7 minutes to do so, after which you will be asked to explain a suitable management plan to the parent.

Examiner's Instructions:

The candidate is a foundation year doctor based at a GP surgery. A parent has made an appointment with the GP to discuss their 24-year-old son called Jacob who has a mild-to moderate learning disability (LD). He has been known and followed up by the LD team since childhood. Recently his parents, who are his carers, have noticed some challenging behaviour. He is not present at this appointment as he is scared of doctors.

The candidate should explore, assess and address the parent's concerns.

Please ask the candidate to explain their management plan to the parent at 7 minutes.

Actor's Instructions:

Background:
You are the parent to Jacob, a 24-year-old man who has a mild-to-moderate learning disability. He has Downs' syndrome. He lives with you and your partner at home and you both share his carer duties. He has been known to the community LD team since childhood. Recently you have noticed some strange and challenging behaviour in John. You are worried that there is an underlying cause.

History of symptoms:
Jacob had a "funny turn" last week at the day centre. The lady at the centre said he may have fainted as they found him on the floor a bit confused. When you picked him up noticed he had wet himself which is abnormal. You have no idea what could be going on. You are very willing to give information but don't know what is useful. Therefore, you wait for the doctor to ask you questions about things.

In the last 6 months you have noticed a change in Jacob. He is usually very affable but has become short tempered and irritable. He has episodes of suddenly lashing out. During these, he will scream, shout and wave his arms around. The last one was 2 weeks ago; he hit your partner in the eye, causing a black eye. He has accidentally hurt himself, banging his head against the wall and causing some scratches on his arm. There seems to be no trigger to this. You have asked him if he is sad about anything but he denies this. He is eating and sleeping normally for him.

Your son has been doing well despite his disabilities. He attended a special school and now attends classes at a local college in computers. He helps out on at your partner's business, with admin and filing work. He really likes this job, but has had to stop due to his unpredictable behaviour. He has friends from a day centre he attends twice a week and will sometimes see these friends socially.

He has a 19-year-old brother, Adam. They spend a lot of time together. Adam has recently moved out of home and bought his own flat in London. He still comes home often but Jacob is missing him.

Jacob once had a bad infection and a temperature which led to a febrile seizure. He went to hospital overnight but then came home. No major health issues since then. He is not on any medication. He does not drink alcohol or take any drugs. He wears glasses but has no other sensory impairments. There have been no psychiatric problems previously. There is a family history of epilepsy, with both your sister and mother having temporal lobe epilepsy.

Questions and actions:
Throughout the consultation: "what could be the cause of his outbursts?", "what happens next?"

OSCE – "Bizarre change in behaviour in Down's syndrome"

Task:	Achieved	Not Achieved
Introduces self		
Clarifies who they are speaking to and who the concern is about		
Establishes rapport		
Elicits history in a concise manner		
Establishes nature of challenging behaviour (duration, course, triggers, previous episodes)		
Explores potential causes sensitively		
Asks about any changes in environment		
Seizures of any sort (duration, what happened during it, tongue biting, incontinence, post-ictal confusion, tonic clonic movements, witnesses statements, evidence of experiencing auras)		
Screen for depression (low mood, anhedonia, fatigue, eating, sleeping)		
Screen for psychotic symptoms (delusions and hallucinations)		
Asks about past medical history		
Asks about medication history, allergies		
Asks about past psychiatric history, learning disability team follow up		
Performs risk assessment: self harm, suicidality & Harm to other people		
Asks about family history of a epilepsy or psychiatric conditions		
Asks about social history (drug, alcohol, smoking and employment)		
Asks about personal history (brief developmental history, birth, school, childhood, relationships)		
Explores parents concerns and fears appropriately		
Creates an appropriate joint management plan to support patient. Including follow up appointment		

to see patient himself & possible other investigates. Asks parent to try to video an episode.		
Recognizes that there is evidence this could be epilepsy. Safety net provided to call ambulance if episode lasts more than 5 minutes.		
Examiner's Global Mark	/5	
Actor / Helper's Global Mark	/5	
Total Station Mark	/30	

Learning Points:

- Epilepsy may be misdiagnosed in patients with learning disability (LD), particularly when there is a history of sudden unexplained aggression, self-mutilation, and other bizarre behaviours. These may include abnormal or stereotyped movements, fixed staring, rapid eye blinking, exaggerated startle, reflex, attention deficits, or unexplained intermittent lethargy.

-

- There are many causes of challenging behaviour in people with LD which must be ruled out (psychiatric disorder, physical health disorder, side effects of medication, environmental changes, sensory deficits, psychosocial factors such as bereavement or disrupted family, recent stressful events, adverse experiences such as social rejection, neglect, physical, emotional or sexual abuse).

- Useful advice when counselling someone who may have a new, or speculative, diagnosis of epilepsy includes to ask a relative to video the episode, and clear safety netting of what to do if it happens again or lasts more than 5 minutes. Strictly speaking, if you are suspecting a new diagnosis of epilepsy, they should be advised not to take baths, perform watersports or drive, until a definitive diagnosis is made.

5.6 "Aggression in Down's Syndrome"

Candidate's Instructions:

A 46-year-old man called Derek attends the GP surgery, he appears to be distressed and is upsetting patients in the waiting room.

You are the foundation doctor working at the practice and have been asked to perform a full Mental State Examination (MSE). Please do not take a history.

You have 6 minutes to perform the MSE, after which you will be asked to present you're your findings, and provide an initial management plan to your supervising GP.

Examiner's Instructions:

A 46-year-old man called Derek has presented to the GP surgery, he appears to be distressed and is upsetting patients in the waiting room.

The foundation doctor working at the practice has been asked to perform a Mental State Examination (MSE).

At 6 minutes ask the candidate the following questions:

1. QUESTION: Please present the MSE
2. QUESTION: Please explain your initial management plan

Actor's Instructions:

Background

You are a 46-year-old man called Derek, and you are angry that you have had to wait all morning for an appointment. You have Down's syndrome and your carer was not able to come with you to the GP as he was unwell this morning. You are distressed that you have been left alone. You have come in to discuss the anti-depressants your GP started you on a month ago. If asked you do not remember the name or the dose of the medication, just that it's a tablet your carer gives you every morning.

This is a MSE station, so the candidate should not be focusing on a detailed history; if they ask, you have hearing problems and wear a hearing aid. You have no known allergies.

Your Mental State:

MSE component	Description
Appearance and Behaviour	Your clothes do not match and are messy. You are agitated, rocking backwards and forwards, and refuse to speak to the doctor, stating that 'you are not my regular doctor'. You eventually agree to see the doctor. You are still angry saying "I had to wait 3 hours for an appointment with my regular doctor and that is not you!" people in the waiting room were staring at you and this made you upset. Your arms are crossed. You initially refuse to answer questions, and are difficult when the doctor asks you personal questions. You put your head in your hands a lot as explaining things is difficult.
Speech	Your speech is slow, and if the doctor speaks quickly or with jargon you do not understand you ask them to repeat or talk slowly.
Mood	You are feeling low in mood and anxious to see a doctor, saying: "my carer has left me ALL alone doctor." Your sleep has improved and are eating more, talk to the doctor about your favourite kinds of food.

Thought	Your thoughts are clear and logical, but you become easily very frustrated. "Come on! You have my records; it is difficult to talk about." Process - repetitive ideas, sometimes going around in circles. You are fixated on medication and bring the topic of conversation back to this if it changes; you have heard of different names and ask the doctor "can't I have that one beginning with P? Or the one beginning with M?" "I don't want to take this medication!" Content –You have been feeling low since you had to move into sheltered accommodation, as your mother was no longer able to take care of you at home. You are feeling better since starting medication (sertraline), but you forgot to take it this morning when your carer did not come. This has caused you a lot of anxiety. You have had problems with depression in the past but this is the first time you have been given medication. You have not had any side effects. You want to come off the medication as you don't like taking pills, you become upset if they suggest that you should stay on medication. You volunteer at the local garden project, if asked about suicidal ideas, you do not understand and have never tried to harm or kill yourself.
Perception	You deny any illusions or visual distortions. You are not hearing voices or seeing anything abnormal. You are not responding to stimuli.
Cognition	You are not confused, but very frustrated. You know where you are, what time it is and who you are. You become even more frustrated at these "silly" questions.
Insight	Being on medication makes you feel very stressed and ideally you don't want to take anything.
Risk	You have not had any suicidal ideation.

AGGRESSION IN DOWNS SYNDROME OSCE – Downs syndrome

Task:	Achieved	Not Achieved
Introduces self		
Confirms patient identity and gains consent		
Asks about presenting complaint		
Apologises for delay in seeing patient		
Comments on appearance– kempt, dishevelled, cleanliness, appropriate clothing for situation		
Comments on behaviour - agitated, calm, aggressive, anxious, eye contact, engagement		
Comments on speech– quality, rate, tone, quantity		
Comments on objective mood – low, euthymic, elated		
Comments on affect – reactive, flat		
Comments on subjective mood – sad, suicidal, hopeless		
Enquires specifically about suicidal thoughts and risk		
Comments on thought form - flight of ideas, circumstantiality		
Comments on thought content - delusions, obsessions, overvalued ideas), thought insertion, withdrawal or broadcast		
Comments on visual hallucinations		
Comments on auditory hallucinations		
Comments on cognition–time, place and person		
Comments on level of insight– ability to recognize problem and necessity of treatment		

QUESTION: Summarises MSE concisely		
QUESTION: Discusses initial management plan: conservative therapies – follow up appointment with regular doctor, contact with carer to arrange appointments, medical management – continue antidepressants		
Non judgmental approach		
Examiner's Global Mark	/5	
Actor / Helper's Global Mark	/5	
Total Station Mark	/30	

Learning Points

- When seeing an angry or agitated patient give them space to air their grievances and apologise early on for any problems that might have been caused.

- When taking a history from someone with learning difficulties, try to avoid any jargon and ask open questions. It is preferable to have a family member or carer present as they know the patient and their habits better

- When assessing someone who is on anti-depressants, remember to reassess for suicidal ideation and depressive symptoms especially in the period following medication initiation. It might be necessary to increase the dose, change the antidepressant or add in another medication to augment the therapy.

Printed in Great Britain
by Amazon

62449060R00200